On Learning
to Heal

CRITICAL GLOBAL HEALTH: Evidence, Efficacy, Ethnography
*A series edited by Vincanne Adams and João Biehl*

# On Learning to Heal

OR,

## WHAT MEDICINE DOESN'T KNOW

ED COHEN

Duke University Press  *Durham and London*  2023

© 2023 DUKE UNIVERSITY PRESS All rights reserved
Printed in the United States of America on acid-free paper ∞
Project editor: Lisa Lawley
Designed by Courtney Leigh Richardson
Typeset in Garamond Premier Pro by Westchester Publishing Services

Library of Congress Cataloging-in-Publication Data
Names: Cohen, Ed, [date] author.
Title: On learning to heal : or, what medicine doesn't know / Ed Cohen.
Other titles: What medicine doesn't know | Critical global health.
Description: Durham : Duke University Press, 2023. | Series: Critical
global health: evidence, efficacy, ethnography | Includes bibliographical
references and index.
Identifiers: LCCN 2022028097 (print)
LCCN 2022028098 (ebook)
ISBN 9781478019329 (PAPERBACK)
ISBN 9781478016670 (hardcover)
ISBN 9781478023944 (ebook)
Subjects: LCSH: Cohen, Ed, 1958– | Mental healing. | Mind and body. |
Healing—Philosophy. | Self-care, Health. | Crohn's disease—Alternative
treatment. | Crohn's disease—Patients. | BISAC: HEALTH & FITNESS /
Diseases & Conditions / General | SOCIAL SCIENCE / Gender Studies
Classification: LCC RZ401 .C646 2023 (print) | LCC RZ401 (ebook) |
DDC 615.8/51—dc23/eng/20220802
LC record available at https://lccn.loc.gov/2022028097
LC ebook record available at https://lccn.loc.gov/2022028098

Cover art: Rod of Asclepius, Wikimedia Commons.

Oh, my body, make of me a man who always questions!
—FRANTZ FANON, *Black Skin, White Masks* (1967 [1952])

"Free Your Mind and Your Ass Will Follow"
—GEORGE CLINTON (1970)

To those from whom I have ever learned anything,
with my deepest gratitude

# Contents

FOUR

When We Learn to Heal, It Matters

121

Coda: Healing with COVID, or Why Medicine Is Not Enough

161

Notes

163

Bibliography

195

Index

211

*Prologue: Invoking Healing*

One must not forget that recovery is brought about not by the physician, but by the sick man himself. He heals himself, by his own power, exactly as he walks by means of his own power, or eats, thinks, breathes, and sleeps.—GEORG GRODDECK, *The Book of the It*, LETTER 32

Much of *On Learning to Heal* was written during the first year and a half of the SARS-CoV-2/COVID-19 pandemic. This coincidence made me acutely aware that neither the word nor the concept of healing (if not the process itself) seemed especially relevant to how we think about this catastrophic event. While politicians and public health officials did not hesitate to recruit war imagery to describe the pandemic—whether characterizing the virus as "the enemy" or representing the scenes in hospitals as "battlefields"—almost no one seemed to consider that healing might offer another possible way to think about our situation. Certainly, media reports assiduously chronicled the heroic efforts by health care providers to support those severely afflicted with the symptoms propagated by the novel (and probably zoonotic) coronavirus. Indeed, during the first months of the COVID-19 pandemic, choruses of clapping, cheering, drumming, and trumpeting regularly started every evening at 7 p.m. in recognition and appreciation of these efforts, not only in my Brooklyn neighborhood but in neighborhoods around the world. This daily anthem offered a sonic tribute to those who toiled, often in underequipped and overcrowded circumstances, to keep the people most afflicted by the effects of SARS-CoV-2 infections alive.

I live around the corner from a large hospital, run by one of New York's major hospital corporations, so it seemed fitting that my neighbors exuberantly expressed their appreciation for the "frontline workers" we saw coming and going past the refrigerated morgue trucks. This sonic ritual, echoed across the globe, recognized in a mundane way something that actually goes on all the time, albeit not always with the same degree of public appreciation: very sick people who require support to go on living receive the active attention of others—at least if it's available and they can afford it. In the case of COVID-19, these acts of attention appeared especially courageous, not only because a deluge of critically ill people, each one a potential vector for the highly contagious virus, easily overwhelmed hospitals but also because so little was known either about the virus or about how to treat it. As medical personnel struggled—frequently without proper personal protective equipment—to improvise new ways to respond to the multiple life-threatening impairments that can follow a SARS-CoV-2 infection, they valiantly exposed themselves to the viral contagion in the service of caring for others whose lives hung in the balance.

However, as much as these efforts deserve our gratitude and respect, something else very important to sustaining life—indeed, something without which no life would ever be sustained—goes unnoticed when we focus our praise exclusively on those who staff our hospitals, no matter how courageous they may be. The fact is that every single person who has contracted COVID-19 and recovered, no matter how much medical intervention they benefited from, has done so because they have an intrinsic capacity to heal. As Georg Groddeck reminded us in the early years of modern medicine, before almost any of its currently effective protocols existed, if we heal, we do the healing, even if we depend on others to assist us. Yet this healing capacity has remained almost entirely unnoticed and unacknowledged in our thinking about the pandemic. Healing is one of the essential tendencies of all living organisms, and without it none of us would still be alive. Unfortunately, when we focus so intently on medicine as a (potentially) curative technology, we often neglect to acknowledge that all medicine can ever do is support and encourage this vital potential. Medicine does not and cannot heal us. Skilled care provided by clinicians, nurses, radiologists, lab workers, respiratory therapists, physical therapists, dialysis technicians, nursing assistants, dieticians, porters, cleaners, and so on, no doubt maintains and sustains the lives of many critically ill patients, including those struggling with COVID-19-related symptoms. Yet it is important to remember: healing doesn't actually travel from the outside in, because whatever can be done *to* us depends on the potential to heal that lives *within* us. Others can support and encourage this capacity, but they do not and cannot make it happen. Of course, because there were no specific treatments for the new disease at the time, those caring for people with COVID justifiably deserve our highest esteem. Still, even given these trying circumstances, healing itself might deserve some praise as well—which is what this book tries to give it.

## Acknowledgments

It took a lot of learning and a lot of healing to write this book on learning to heal—which is just another way of saying it required a lot of encouragement and support. If I've learned anything from this project, it's that although learning and healing constitute tendencies to which we can aspire, they aren't certainties by any stretch of the imagination. That's why we need other people to keep us tending in the right direction. Fortunately for me, I had a lot of help staying on track.

This book would not exist without what I have learned from my beloved teachers: Rachel Remen, Emilie Conrad, Susan Harper, Carol Joyce, Mary Swanson, and Mayla Riley. From each of you I learned how to stay rooted and grow strong—if not wise—at the same time. You each helped me cultivate vital energies that I didn't even know existed, and I bow in gratitude to your wisdom and your love.

My extended pod created a nourishing context in which I could ruminate on healing as well as heal, never an easy task, especially in the midst of the COVID-19 pandemic. Their ongoing enthusiasm for this project made it possible to finally finish even when it looked like we might all be going to hell in a handcart. Big props to Emma Bianchi, Ellen Bruno, Maria Damon, David Eng, David Kazanjian, Michael Lighty, Ardele Lister, Rebecca Mark, Jennie Portnof, Teemu Ruskola, Josie Saldana, and Caroline Streeter for all the love and laughs.

Special thanks to Julie Livingston, who has always been my ideal reader for this book, the perfect IBD companion, and my baking buddy; Cathy Davidson, who saved me from a really shitty title and helped me see why the book deserved better; and Joan Scott, whose enthusiasm and sage advice helped me find my way into nerd-vana.

I am exceedingly grateful to the many people who read and commented on drafts of this project along the way: Emma Bianchi, Maria Damon, David Eng, Simon Goldin, Eben Kirksey, David Kazanjian, Ardele Lister, Julie Livingston, Rebecca Mark, Fareen Parvez, Jennie Portnof, Sarah Quinn, Teemu Ruskola, Josie Saldana, Gayle Solomon, Latif Tas, and the anonymous readers for Duke University Press. I also benefited enormously from the sage editorial direction provided by David Lobenstine and the aptly named Laura Helper. Your thoughtful insights and reflections have improved this text enormously—and made it considerably more readable.

Because spending hours and hours hunched over a computer has never been very healing for any body, I have been very fortunate to have genius somatics practitioners who have helped bend me back into shape. Major thanks to Marcelo Coutinho, Ariel Kiley, Joe Spilone, and Farrel Duncan for helping me recover from writing this book on a regular basis.

My 2019–20 fellows at the Institute for Advanced Studies in Princeton were wonderful thinking companions, and I am deeply grateful to Didier Fassin and Alondra Nelson for inviting me for the year—alas, sadly abbreviated by COVID-19. Also, big thanks to Elspeth Brown and Eva-Lynn Jagoe for organizing the workshop in nonacademic writing for academics at the University of Toronto, and all the participants—especially Ann Cvetkovitch—for teaching me to think critically about my narrative voice, which turned out to be what I most needed to learn about writing in order to write this book.

Thanks to Ken Wissoker for including me in Duke's impeccably curated list. It's an honor to appear in such great company again. Thank you to all the people at Duke who make such beautiful books (and make making them so easy on their authors): Ryan Kendall for facilitating the curation process; Lisa Lawley for masterfully overseeing the production; Courtney Leigh Richardson for such a beautiful cover and wonderful layout, and for graciously accepting the rod of Asclepius as a design constraint; and the aptly named Laura Sell for helping disseminate this book as widely as possible.

And in memoriam: to Chunky and Monkey, whose feline love kept my lap warm throughout this project.

*A Note on Shit*

This book uses the word *shit* an inordinate number of times. Some people may find that troubling. To them I apologize in advance and as consolation offer the following insight gathered from the French philosophers Gilles Deleuze and Félix Guattari: "Only the mind is capable of shitting."[1]

# Overture

## HEALING AS DESIRE AND VALUE

Knowledge does not necessarily emanate from transcendence . . . but from concatenations of the imaginary and desires.—HENRI ATLAN, "Knowledge of Ignorance" (2011)

When I might have needed it most, I had no idea that something like healing could happen. Indeed, I might never have known about healing if it hadn't bitten me in the ass. After I was diagnosed with Crohn's disease at the age of thirteen, I assumed that I would always bear its stigmata. My doctors told me that there was no cure for Crohn's and that probably the best I could hope for was to manage my symptoms medically for the rest of my life. If I were lucky, they said, I might experience periods of remission but I could never expect it to go away entirely. Alas, I wasn't so lucky. Instead of experiencing remissions, over time my symptoms just got worse. I lived with this bleak prognosis for over a decade, and it thoroughly infected my youthful fantasies about the future—not in a good way. Then, in my early twenties, I got really sick and almost died. But miraculously, I didn't, and afterward I actually started getting better. This entirely unexpected turn of events, which I recount in the following chapters, animates the deep appreciation for healing that inspires this book. Healing came to me unbidden, because I had no idea that I could call upon it, let alone how I might do that. I certainly never imagined that I could learn to heal or that learning had anything to do with healing. Yet when I felt its first sparks ignite in me while lying on my bed in the ICU, healing definitely caught my attention. Months afterward, when I had recovered enough physically, though not yet psychically or spiritually, I started to realize that in order to tend the flame those sparks had ignited, I would need to learn both to desire healing and to value it—something I've been trying to do for the last four decades. This book traces that learning curve.

During the most acute phase of my illness, chronicled in chapter 1, I spent several months in Stanford University Hospital. After my release, I attempted to go back to life as I had known it. I was a graduate student at the time, living with others from my cohort in a collective house in Palo Alto. A friend of mine, Gonzalo, was living on his own across town in a little cottage on Perry Lane. Tom Wolfe had made Perry Lane famous in *The Electric Kool-Aid Acid Test* as "Arcadia just off the edge of Stanford golf course." In the early 1960s, Ken Kesey wrote *One Flew over the Cuckoo's Nest* in one of the small cabins that lined the street, and it soon became renowned as an enclave for the gestating '60s counterculture as well as the epicenter of the early LSD experiences that soon took America by storm. By the time Gonzalo rented one of the Perry Lane shacks in 1982, that scene was long gone, but its vibrations definitely lingered, even without the psychedelics. Because he was going to visit his family in Peru over Christmas vacation, Gonzalo offered me the place in his absence. This would be my first chance to spend any time alone since my extended hospital odyssey, and I relished the idea of having a bit of solitude to reflect on what I'd just been through. Needless to say, when you're critically ill in the hospital, there isn't much solitude, let alone space for reflection.

During my first few days on Perry Lane, I grooved in a nice rhythm, waking up at midday and then drinking two cups of tea and eating three pieces of Ryvita with peanut butter and apricot jam while sitting on the back steps. (I still have this breakfast around noon every day—often sitting in my garden—which is why I can remember it.) Reading. Getting a little stoned. Listening to music. Taking a bike ride through the back streets of Menlo Park. Napping. Having a late afternoon snack. And then, just before sunset, wandering along the Arcadian paths between Perry Lane and Stanford's golf course. Trees have always embraced me. I grew up in a small town in northern Maryland, which was incredibly lush, and our house was completely sheltered by trees. A towering sycamore erupted from the middle of our driveway, and a magnificent five-trunked maple behind the house hosted our forts and secret clubs. Beyond the cow pasture that abutted our yard was a little wood with a stream running through it, where we would hunt for frogs and crayfish. From an early age, trees offered me refuge when I needed it. They were my friends. So when I needed to find myself again after my return to the land of the living, the trees at the end of Perry Lane beckoned me.

One evening as I was making my way through these woods, I was suddenly stopped in my tracks. My feet seemingly had rooted into the soil, and something vital was flowing up into me from the earth. At first I felt a deep stillness, as if all sound had fallen away, but then something shifted. It wasn't as if I heard someone speaking, but I apprehended a very clear message that seemed channeled by the trees. It wasn't in words exactly, but I couldn't mistake the meaning: either I could keep following the path I'd been on since my diagnosis a decade earlier, which would only lead me back through acute illness—and perhaps again to near-death—or I could learn new ways to live. Even though the notion that trees could directly communicate wisdom violated every precept I had been brought up to believe, I immediately understood that I needed to pay attention to this message.

Obviously, I knew trees can't actually talk to people, yet I had no idea where the message could have come from except from the trees. I no longer question the wisdom of trees. In fact, I often tell my students the story of the Buddha's enlightenment under the Bodhi tree, where—as all the forces of illusion arrayed against him threatening him with annihilation—he simply turned his thumb down to touch the earth without breaking his meditation and called upon it to witness his right to exist. Instantly, all illusions vanished and the Buddha achieved enlightenment. Where do you think he learned that, I ask my students, except from the Bodhi tree, which had been whispering in his ear all along as he sat beneath it? Some people say that trees are the most spiritual beings because they give so unstintingly of themselves. I don't know if that's true, though it seems likely; what I do know is that standing in the middle of those trees that evening, I realized that something in me knew how to heal and that if I didn't want to keep living from one crisis to the next, I'd need to learn to cultivate that capacity.

None of my myriad medical encounters had prepared me for this epiphany. Au contraire, medicine's genius lay in keeping me alive, in helping me sustain myself in the midst of a chronic condition that it had no means to heal, let alone cure. In fact, healing never figured into the picture my doctors sketched for me about the probable trajectory of my disease's progression. Thus, they had no explanations for why I had swerved so precipitously away from death, so soon after I had swerved so perilously close to it. Yet the trees seemed quite emphatic that they had important insights to offer on this point, and I can retrospectively affirm that they knew what they were talking about! Once I started to take their message to heart, my life began to change rapidly. I began to discover teachers about whom I'd previously had no inkling and toward whom I probably would have had no inclination but who, once I encountered them, helped me learn to heal more consciously and consistently. This book honors those teachers by trying to disseminate the seeds of their teachings as they have grown within me. Indeed, through these encounters, I gradually began to discern that healing, learning, and growing are all vital values, essential to life, and that they matter deeply, whether we realize it or not.

For many years, when I thought back to this inflection point in my illness narrative, I wondered why the trees had been so wise in this regard and why they had spoken to me. Only in the process of writing this book did a satisfactory answer present itself. In her memoir *God's Hotel*, the physician and historian of medicine Victoria Sweet suggested something that I'd never considered.[1] She tells the story of an acutely ill patient, Terry, a homeless Native American woman who was a sex worker and heroin addict, whose "miraculous healing" dramatically changed Sweet's ideas about how she practiced medicine. Although many doctors have witnessed such dramatic and improbable recoveries, most probably don't dwell on the inexplicable transformations that occasionally occur before their eyes. Even their astonishment in the face of such occurrences doesn't often revise their medical perspective. However, Sweet's did, by viewing Terry's recovery through the perspective of a twelfth-century German mystic, theologian, musician, and medical practitioner, Hildegard of Bingen. Hildegard first came into Sweet's life by way of a book that Sweet stumbled upon while searching for answers to questions about life and death that arose from her encounters with patients but for which her modern medical training had unfortunately not prepared her. Despite the extreme divergence between Hildegard's medieval mystical methods and Sweet's bioscientifically based education, she recognized something within Hildegard's orientation that enabled her to engage more effectively with the suffering of those who sought her help. Captivated by Hildegard's ethos, Sweet eventually undertook a PhD in the history of medicine, writing a dissertation on Hildegard and premodern medicine that became the basis for a wonderful book, *Rooted in the Earth, Rooted in the Sky*.

Eight centuries before modern medicine, Sweet tells us, Hildegard wrote two manuscripts, *Physica* and *Causae et Curae*, that compiled her wisdom about medical practice. The medicine of Hildegard's period was humoral, derived from ancient Greek and Roman thinking and based on a system of elements (earth, water, fire, air), qualities (hot, dry, wet, cold), and humors (blood, phlegm, black bile, and yellow bile), whose balances and imbalances ruled the conditions of living bodies.[2] While Hildegard largely adhered to this framework, Sweet recognized another germinal element in Hildegard's writings that augmented her canonical humoralism. For, in addition to her spiritual and medical perspectives, which she always wove together, Hildegard evinced a reverence for the wisdom of plants. Given her context, this was not entirely surprising. Hildegard not only lived in an agrarian culture, in which daily life revolved around the natural cycles of cultivation, growth, and harvest, but she was also a healer-gardener, growing and tending much of the pharmacopoeia that she employed. Thus, in both her medical and mystical writings, she evoked a concept, *viriditas*, derived from the Latin *viridis*, meaning green, fresh, blooming, vigorous, verdant, abounding in green growth.[3] *Viriditas* for Hildegard indicated a state of greenness or "greening," and Sweet suggests that it might have represented "a precedent in older medical texts for a power related to plants that also stood for the body's ability to heal."[4]

Hildegard didn't invent *viriditas*. The concept had appeared both in Aristotelian natural philosophy about plants and in earlier Christian spiritual writings, but she adapted it to different ends. Taking the plant world for inspiration, Hildegard recognized an essential affinity between the vitality of living plant bodies and that of animal bodies. On one hand, this affinity made sense given the use of herbal remedies, which constituted a major part of the medieval pharmacopoeia. Plant medicine spoke directly to the *viriditas* in humans and encouraged its efflorescence. On the other, *viriditas* figured as a force that animated bodies, infusing them with vigor, health, and fertility. As Sweet describes it, for Hildegard, *viriditas* contained "both substance and power."[5] In this sense, it resonated with other concepts familiar to medieval medicine: *humidium radicale* (which Sweet describes as "radical moisture," the "'root,' or basic moisture from which a life begins"), *calor inatus* (the "inborn heat" that "provided the power for growth and maturation"), and the *vis medicatrix naturae* (the healing power of nature, akin to the Greek *phusis*, which invoked "the body's innate vigor or strength, the inborn power of the live body to maintain its integrity"). Yet, more than any one of them, for Hildegard *viriditas* encompassed all these possibilities, Sweet argues, because both plants and animals "were rooted in the same earth and subject to the same sky."

Needless to say, the convergence between Hildegard's orientation and Sweet's own medical practice occurred in a clinical setting where her encounter with Terry's unanticipated if not inexplicable healing revised Sweet's scholarly understanding of Hildegard's teachings. Sharing the story of Terry's recovery, Sweet declares that Terry "would show me what *viriditas* really meant."[6] I can't do justice to Sweet's account, so you should read it for yourself. However, the bare bones (in this case literal) of Terry's story should suffice to make the point. No doubt Terry was among the most sexually, racially, and economically vulnerable Americans. She entered Sweet's universe at Laguna Honda Hospital in San Francisco, the last "almshouse in America," while recovering from transverse myelitis, which caused her to lose function of her arms and legs. During her extended rehabilitation, Terry would bounce back and forth between the hospital and the streets, abetted by her abusive boyfriend and her drug habit, each time returning in a more and more debilitated state. Eventually she developed a bedsore on her back that ripened into a festering open wound which threatened her life. Here's Sweet's description:

> Terry's bedsore was scary. She had no protection. Everything delicate and crucial in her body—bones, kidneys, spinal cord—was exposed and vulnerable to an environment full of danger, full of germs—to bacteria of all sorts and from every source, even the bacteria that live on and within our bodies. Giving antibiotics to try to prevent infection wouldn't protect her. I knew because germs would become rapidly resistant to them. And the bedsore was too big to graft, even if the surgeons agreed. It would have to heal on its own and that would take years.[7]

As Sweet suggests, at this point Terry had reached an impasse. Medicine had no more magic bullets to protect her. Either Terry's wound would heal from within, or she would die.

Of course, that didn't mean nothing could be done. As Sweet recounts, what Laguna Honda Hospital could give Terry was ongoing care that would support and encourage her going-on-living as the healing process took place. Sweet describes the gist of this caring as "removing obstructions to *viriditas*," as clearing away the impediments that prevented Terry's healing from flourishing within her.[8] Obviously, one of the main obstructions to her healing was the context in which Terry lived. A homeless, heroin-addicted sex worker living on the streets with an abusive partner doesn't have much that allows *viriditas* to take root. However, in Laguna Honda, where not only were her survival needs satisfied but she received respectful care, Terry's capacity to heal could begin to thrive. Not that it happened all at once. As Sweet explains, this was a long process, over two and a half years, so what Terry's healing also required was the gift of time.

Needless to say, healing is always a temporal process. Healing is a matter of time, and healing makes time matter—in this case quite literally, as Terry's wound gradually healed itself from the inside out, regenerating the cells and tissues whose degeneration and destruction had brought her to the edge of death. However, as Sweet emphasizes, Terry's healing didn't only entail physiology. During the process, she was able to break up with her abusive partner, detox from her drug and nicotine use, and finally, when she was well enough, reunite with a brother from whom she'd been estranged, who took her in and assumed responsibility for her care. In Terry's case, Sweet shows, removing the obstacles to *viriditas*, tending and cultivating its potency, worked miracles, albeit slow ones.[9] It allowed the *vis medicatrix naturae* to manifest because it mattered. In Sweet's gloss, the *vis medicatrix naturae* doesn't simply mean the power of nature to heal us; rather, she suggests that it really names "'the remedying force of your own nature to be itself,' to turn back into itself when it has been wounded."[10]

The greening force of *viriditas*, along with the healing force of the *vis medicatrix*, gestures toward possibilities that modern medicine seems to have forgotten. Yet all of its efforts depend upon these forgotten and often neglected possibilities. Healing manifests itself all around us if we have eyes to see and minds to care. For example, Sweet's descriptions of Terry's healing wounds remind me of trees I have known. Despite lightning strikes, tornadoes, uprootings, fungal blights, and so on, trees can continue to grow, putting forth new shoots and leaves, filling in gaps in their own crowns as they reach toward the sun. Lost branches can resolve into scars. Cancers can exude as bulbous cankers. If a tree is well rooted, new growth can spring forth even when the main trunk is lost, as when logged old-growth redwoods send up fairy rings of progeny around an absent center. Healing, like growth and development, and perhaps like evolution, represents a natural propensity for all life. As modern humans we may no longer acknowledge this fact as much as we should, but that need not stymie our efforts. After all, among our many attributes, as humans we excel at learning, so perhaps we might simply need to make more effort to learn to desire and value healing in order to learn to heal.

*On Learning to Heal* seeks to revive our appreciation for healing not only as a natural resource but as a vital value, which for humans means a political and economic value as well as a biological one. Biologically speaking, to recognize healing as a value simply means that an organism takes its going-on-living as significant. Or, as Friedrich Nietzsche put it with his typical diagnostic power: "The standpoint of 'value' is the standpoint of conditions of preservation and enhancement for complex forms of relative life duration within the flux of becoming."[11] Disease and injury are always meaningful for a living organism. They represent challenges to vital functions that call an organism's living—or at least

its mode of living—into question. Thus, insofar as any life form tends, or intends, to go on living, healing partakes of the imperative that the seventeenth-
century philosopher Baruch Spinoza called *conatus*.[12] In his *Ethics*, Spinoza
defined *conatus* as a "striv[ing] to persevere in . . . being," where this striving
represented "the actual essence of the being."[13] For Spinoza, *conatus* pertained
to all beings, whether animate or inanimate. He held that all being is one—
including God and nature—and objected to the pretension that humans are
exceptional beings, as if we constitute a "kingdom within a kingdom."[14] This
is probably also the case for all living beings. Life is not its own dominion, especially if biology continues geology by other means—as the Russian geologist/
geochemist Vladimir Vernadsky argued and as global warming now confirms.[15]
Yet, even so, animate beings express greater degrees of indetermination than inanimate ones. That is to say, while animate and inanimate beings always remain
deeply entangled, animate beings multiply the range of variables with which
they can engage, and these variations introduce more possibilities for how they
interact with inanimate beings as well as other animate ones. As Henri Bergson
put it, "The role of life is to insert some indetermination into matter. Indeterminate, i.e., unforeseeable, are the forms it creates in the course of its evolution.
More and more indeterminate also, more and more free."[16]

Such unforeseeable possibilities introduce an element of choice or decision
for living beings that, as far as we know, does not pertain to the nonliving.
And whenever decisions enter into consideration—even when they remain
nonconscious—they introduce occasions for judgment. Living beings must
orient themselves toward or away from this or that vital variable (e.g., toward
food, away from toxins; toward prey, away from predators), and these orientations necessarily require some criteria for evaluation. Such criteria, which seek
to enhance an organism's going-on-being, are what we call values. Thus, it's no
coincidence that our word *value* comes from a Latin term, *valere*, which means
to be physically powerful or strong, have strength, have strength or wellness,
be in sound health.[17] At its most basic—and most abstract—life is a value that
manifests values because the going-on-living of any life form entails a decisive
orientation toward those possibilities that enable it to persevere in its being.[18]

At a fundamental level, healing names an essential reparative capability that
all organisms, including trees and humans, need to realize in order to go on
living. Yet for humans, healing, like any vital value, also takes on other implications insofar as we can reflect upon them. As the historian, philosopher, and
physician Georges Canguilhem reminds us, "The living human body is the
totality of powers of an existent that has the capacity to evaluate and represent these powers to itself, their exercise and their limits."[19] The value contexts

that humans create expand the domains of possible interaction between the animate and inanimate. While other species always manifest values in their lives insofar as they go on living—hence, plants orient themselves toward the sun (heliotropism); bacteria orient themselves toward or away from chemical gradients (chemotaxis); and predatory animals orient themselves toward prey (predation)—we humans seem to expand our modes of valuation beyond our mere subsistence. As Alfred North Whitehead characterized it, our vital imperative as humans impels us "(1) to live; (2) to live well; (3) to live better."[20] Needless to say, this motive requires making choices that shape not just the fact of our living, but also the manner in which we live. Furthermore, directed by this impulse, we also establish modes of living that vary across time and place.

To speak of healing as a desire and a value, then, is to recognize not only that as humans we manifest an intrinsic potential for subsisting, for going on living, but that we can also cultivate a capacity for living in more life-enhancing ways. Ideally, this might be what politics and economics attempt to do. By focusing our attention and directing our decisions, our values can enable us to create new modes of living, to which we can aspire, because we desire to live otherwise than we currently do or can. And because as humans we always live both individually and collectively, these vital decisions—whether biological, political, or economic, if we can even distinguish these anymore—increasingly ask us to realize that healing represents a desirable value.

Alas, because our culture has largely neglected the value of healing, many of us don't recognize it as such. That was certainly my experience. *On Learning to Heal* chronicles the long and challenging process through which I learned both to desire healing and to heal—and perhaps learning to desire healing is itself a form of healing, or at least a step in that direction. By allowing myself to desire to heal, I began to learn to heal even as I learned that healing also entails embracing the possibility for growing and developing. Healing, growing, developing, learning, and evolving are often braided together. They all constitute vital values that can prompt us to extend our existence beyond subsistence, to desire that our lives might concern more than merely going-on-living. How this desire moves (in) us cannot be determined in advance because, like living, healing is an ongoing process—until it's not.

The subtitle of this book is *What Medicine Doesn't Know*. I mean no disrespect to medicine by pointing out that, by and large, medicine underappreciates what Henri Atlan calls our "knowledge of ignorance." In a short essay with this title,

Atlan, a philosopher trained in biophysics and medicine, brings his admiration for Spinoza's ethics to bear on his work as a bioscientist. Atlan's intent in this piece is clear: to remind those who practice science and especially bioscience (as well as those of us who rely on their insights) that while these practices are powerful and important, they remain limited both in principle and in fact. Addressing the restrictions that underwrite scientific and bioscientific practice, Atlan informs us that "today's science restricts itself to the enormous domain within which it is increasingly preoccupied with mastering artifacts born in the laboratories for the sole purpose of being mastered."[21] Indeed, the possibility of artifactually restricting "life" to the confines of a laboratory constitutes the condition of possibility for all contemporary bioscience and biomedicine.[22] (The apotheosis of "laboratory life" occurs in synthetic biology, which aims to create new, "better designed," forms of life.[23]) The results of such artifactual manipulation have certainly proved astonishingly effective, yielding life-saving and life-extending technologies and treatments unimaginable before the invention of the knowledge domain now claimed by the life sciences. Yet their very successes often tend to obscure their intrinsic limitations. Atlan, following Spinoza, recalls these limitations, not in order to diminish the significance of bioscientific insights, but in order to put them into perspective—a perspective that conceives knowledge in *and as* life.

If, as Michel Foucault admonishes us, "to form concepts is one way of living, not of killing life," Atlan places the production of bioscientific concepts within the limits that life imposes upon us.[24] In other words, he stresses that as living beings we can only ever apprehend a limited range of the phenomena that determine our lives: "our ignorance of the *totality* of determinations is part of natural reality *as much as the determinations themselves* because this ignorance produces effects—our behavior—different from what they would be if we had total knowledge of natural determinations. . . . Our ignorance of the totality of determinations is equivalent, *insofar as it matters to us*, to the *real* existence of indeterminations in nature."[25] In the medical arena, acknowledging the indeterminacy of knowledge as a real limit proves especially challenging because, when we approach medicine, we often desire not only that medicine knows what is wrong with us but also that it knows how to rectify this wrongness. However, our desires do not always correspond to our possibilities. Atlan emphasizes the limits of our capacity to know in order to remind us that our knowledge arises only within the ambit of our existence as living beings. In other words, knowledge cannot encompass the totality of our lives because it is at best partial (in all senses). Thus, it is also crucial to remember, as Atlan admonishes us, that "our behavior can be directed only *both by what we know of our determinations and by the fact that we know we don't know everything.*[26]

My belated gratitude for Atlan's insight stems from my willful ignorance of my own ignorance. When I first entered the medical labyrinth devoted to the diagnosis and treatment of Crohn's disease, I had an overwhelming desire that my doctors know what was wrong with me. Of course, in some sense they did, because they were eventually able to correlate my symptoms with a recognizable category of pathology and to prescribe a powerful pharmacological regime that would suppress some of its more dire symptoms, at least for a while. However, in a larger sense, I would later come to learn, they didn't know that much at all. The causes of Crohn's disease, like all of the sixty to eighty other diseases considered to have autoimmune etiologies, remain elusive. Moreover, why Crohn's occurs, when it occurs, to those in whom it occurs, completely exceeds biomedical explanation. Again, this statement is not meant to impugn the knowledge that biomedicine does engender but rather to put it into another perspective—the perspective of a person diagnosed with this disease who has lived with it for almost half a century.

For the first decade or so of my life with Crohn's, I thoroughly imbibed the medical explanations for my illness. At the time of my diagnosis, I was given a very basic explanation of what Crohn's entailed from a gastroenterological point of view. I was told I had an autoimmune disorder and that I needed to take drugs that would tamp down my body's immune responses to my own tissues, which in my case primarily affected the lining of my small intestine. Because I didn't know enough to question this way of thinking, I took it on faith and relied on the treatments presented to me as if they constituted the entirety of available therapeutic possibilities. Hence, along with the pills my doctors prescribed, I also ingested their ways of thinking about my condition, as if their knowledge represented my truth.

Obviously, medicine doesn't oblige us to take its insights on faith, which is in part why it clings closely to science, whose truths supposedly derive from lab-based facts. Yet, much as medicine may rely on bioscientific knowledge to underwrite its practice, medicine itself is not strictly scientific, let alone a science, despite the recent efforts of evidence-based medicine to assimilate medicine's protocols to more scientific-seeming standards.[27] At some level medicine does know this, even if it consigns this knowledge of its ignorance to the small print as a way of limiting its legal liability. That's why, when I recently had a hip replacement operation, I had to sign a medical consent form that included the following disclaimer: "I understand that medicine is not an exact science." The thing is, while I do understand this, I'm not certain those who act in the name of medicine always do. And in any case, scientific knowledge itself is never transparent to reality, as Atlan underscores: "Without sacrificing any rigor in predicting observable facts, we can choose among different theories the one (or the ones) favoring the norm that suits us. . . . The choice of theory will be an exercise in wishful thinking."[28] Until I started to become aware of the wishful thinking in which modern medicine partakes, I had no way to interrogate the effects of its explanations and therapies on my experiences. However, once I became attuned to thinking of medicine's knowledge as a historical and cultural artifact, itself an effect of the modern imagination more generally, I could begin to question the significance of its many unconscious assumptions.

As often happens to me, my timing in this attunement was both lucky and unfortunate. My most severe Crohn's crisis, as well as my miraculous healing from it, occurred over the spring and summer of 1982 and randomly coincided with the advent of the AIDS epidemic in North America. Thus, while AIDS unfortunately had a profound impact on my life as a young gay man living in San Francisco during the 1980s, it also, luckily for me (as well as for many others), sparked many intense critical reflections on the ways medicine made sense of the emergent pandemic. By 1987, it also gave rise to a political movement, ACT-UP (AIDS Coalition to Unleash Power), that not only recognized that medical knowledge always relies on (often unacknowledged) political assumptions but also demanded that knowledge engendered by people diagnosed as "living with AIDS" be valued as medically relevant.[29] From these historically specific engagements with medicine's limitations, I learned to consider that while biomedicine and bioscience have a panoply of possible resources—although not a monopoly on them—they don't always avail themselves of those resources in optimal ways. Thinking critically about HIV/AIDS not only taught me how to reflect on the values that medicine incorporates within its explanations but also revealed that only by reflecting on these values does it become possible to question the decisions medicine makes on our behalf when it deploys its knowledge to assuage our ills.[30]

Much of this book concerns the backstory of modern medicine. It seeks to disclose the desires and values that medicine incorporates on its way to becoming modern in order to consider whether they are necessary, let alone helpful. In order to do so, it traces one trajectory of thinking and practice that has come to dominate Western understandings of therapeutic action. In particular, it considers moments in medicine's history when certain assumptions about what it means to be a living being become part of medicine's "reason"—in the double sense of its motive and its logic. By exploring these developments in medical thinking, *On Learning to Heal* attempts to illuminate the ways that medicine's investments in *knowing* "what's wrong with us" and how to "fix it" might have unnecessarily and unwittingly discouraged our capacity *to learn* to heal. Indeed, as the rest of the book emphasizes, medicine's insistence that such knowledge constitutes our paramount therapeutic resource is what has made medicine "medicine" ever since it differentiated itself from all other therapeutic practices twenty-five hundred years ago.

As medicine became increasingly accepted as the dominant therapeutic modality in Western cultures, especially over the last century and a half, other ways of assuaging illness came to seem less and less credible to more and more people. Indeed, medical authorities actively demeaned other therapeutic means as part of their market strategy, and it seems to have been extraordinarily successful (increasingly even in cultural contexts in which nonmedical forms of therapeutic intervention had prevailed). In the United States, this included the disparagement not only of nonorthodox or eclectic forms of medicine but also of the therapies developed by indigenous and (formerly) enslaved people as well as those characterized as "women's medicine" or "folk medicine."[31] Certainly, this observation does not diminish the astounding accomplishments of our medical knowledge.[32] Nor does it mean that "medicine" as such constitutes a homogeneous domain. Multiple practical knowledges inform different medical subspecialties; palliative care is different from family medicine is different from oncology is different from psychiatry is different from public health. Nevertheless, insofar as they claim legitimacy as forms of medicine, all these diverse medical practices partake of the same sets of authorization, training, and licensing requirements that instill a commitment to particular ways of knowing as their raison d'être (as chapter 3 elaborates). Paradoxically, however, as the claims made by, for, and upon medical ways of knowing have expanded, medicine's interests in healing, as a general phenomenon intrinsic to all living beings, have radically diminished in favor of concepts like treatment and cure. Moreover, as modern medicine has invented new therapies and technologies capable of modulating organic life at the level of our tissues, cells, and molecules (including the complex crystalline molecule we call DNA), we have tended to forget that these protocols work only insofar as they augment or support our own tendencies to heal at all these levels as well.

Of course, you might wonder: If this is the case, why don't we know it already? Or conversely, why do we give medicine so much credit for our own capacities? Why don't we honor the power to heal that each one of us manifests so long as we go on living? If we are still alive (which, since you're reading this book, I'll assume you are), at some level we do know something about healing. All of us have myriad experiences of healing that we rely on all the time. When we cut a finger, we might disinfect it and put on a bandage, but our finger heals by itself, and not because we have any special knowledge of the biomechanics of tissue repair. The same can be said of any number of mundane experiences that we regularly survive, either with or without medical consultation. These might seem like trivial cases, yet even—or especially—the most intensive and invasive high-tech medical interventions depend on the same healing capacity. For example, when oncologists poison (chemotherapy), slash (surgery), or burn (radiation) us in order to treat cancer, they do so assuming that we have an intrinsic tendency to recover from these therapeutic aggressions.[33] If we didn't, these treatments would kill us, as indeed they sometimes do. Yet, in general, medicine doesn't much concern itself with supporting or encouraging our recovery from such assaults, outsourcing (or offloading?) this responsibility onto other forms of care.[34]

One of the reasons we don't pay as much attention to our own healing capacities as we might—or ought—is that we often rely on medicine to know something about our lives that we don't know ourselves. When we invest medicine with this authority, we can be seduced into thinking not only that it knows more than we do, or that its ways of knowing constitute the only ways of knowing, but also that it addresses the only things worth knowing. Nothing about medicine necessarily demands this compliance from us—although medicine does in fact evaluate patients' responses to prescribed treatments in terms of our compliance with them.[35] In doing so, it asks us to fold or bend with it (which is what *comply* means etymologically), if not to actually bow down before it. Yet, by and large, our compliance does not need to be coerced; much of the time, most of us willingly take what medicine has to offer without compulsion (anti-vaxxers notwithstanding). Insofar as we desire medicine to transform us, we readily take on—and take in—both its ways of knowing and its ways of not-knowing. And, since medicine frequently fails to "know its ignorance," as Atlan puts it, we in turn, with our passionate desires for its knowing ways to work, often fail to know its ignorance as well. However, if we begin to understand how medical knowledge became so compelling in the first place, perhaps we can discover ways to augment this knowledge by learning to attend to and encourage the capacity to heal that lives within us—as long as we're still alive.

To this end, *On Learning to Heal* makes a distinction between knowing and learning. Both are essential to our going-on-living, yet the former can often impede the latter. If you think you already know, you might be less inclined to learn. Conversely, we can learn things that we do not and perhaps cannot know. To take a banal example—which is nonetheless very relevant to my story of living with Crohn's—as infants most of us learn to control our urination and defecation according to culturally prescribed patterns that, since the invention of the utility referred to as the toilet, we call "toilet training."[36] If we do not learn how to do this, or cannot do this, our lives will be severely compromised (as I learned from my extensive experiences with incontinence). Yet we do not necessarily know how we do this. Learning to control our sphincters until we find an appropriate place or time to release them requires incorporating an exquisite ensemble, not only of neuromuscular activities but also of psycho-cultural norms, whose underlying biochemistries and biophysiologies remain partially understood at best. As this mundane yet ubiquitous example demonstrates, knowing and learning can invoke different capacities, and the latter does not always entail the former. Learning to heal does not necessarily require us to know how we heal, but it does require that we desire to heal and that we actively value this possibility. In tracing my own learning curve about healing in this book, I am trying to suggest that when we take medicine's knowing ways for granted, we might unwittingly impede our ability to learn to heal, especially since healing has increasingly been rendered tangential to modern medicine's scientific aspirations.

Needless to say, over the last century and a half, medical knowledge has shored up its bona fides by situating its practice within the purview of science—even while acknowledging (as the consent form I had to sign before my hip surgery affirmed) that it is "not an exact science." Without question, medicine's pursuit of scientific rigor has led to wonderful, previously unimaginable treatment options. And because my own life has been saved by such options a number of times, I am definitely not one to gainsay these achievements. Yet, despite the patently productive alliances between medicine and bioscience, medicine's scientific inclination also introduces a significant problem as well, one that helps explain why healing has become much less central to it.[37]

Science as we know it constitutes itself as an authoritative discourse, that is, one that can legitimately claim to speak the truth, by disqualifying other ways of making sense as less true (if not false). Disqualification provides science with a means of regulating which explanations reside "within the true" and which do not.[38] This boundary maintenance requires that science distinguish between those methods appropriate to producing verifiable knowledge and those that it deems at best unreliable or at worst subjective. As a result, other ways of making sense of the world are discredited, consigned to the realm of fantasy, magical thinking, hype, trickery, bias, and such. By establishing an excluded outside that it sees as beyond the pale, science attempts to purify its own procedures and keep them free of such contamination.[39] Michel Foucault thus describes the way that science seeks to purge the world of "a whole series of knowledges that have been disqualified as non-conceptual knowledges, as insufficiently elaborated knowledges: naïve knowledges, hierarchically inferior knowledges, knowledges that are below the required level of erudition or scientificity."[40] He names these excluded possibilities "subjugated knowledges"—types of knowledge that were banished from the scientific domain of "the true" (e.g., alchemy, witchcraft, spiritualism, herbalism, shamanism, midwifery) and whose exclusion conversely affirms scientific knowledge as true. In relation to modern scientific medicine, acupuncture, chiropractic, homeopathy, osteopathy, Ayurveda, hypnotherapy, bioenergetics, energy balancing, and kinesiology name just some of the monsters that continue to lurk beyond the simultaneously professional and commercial boundaries that scientific medicine establishes.

Nevertheless, such subjugated knowledges contain their own specific logics, languages, and efficacies, some of which have persistently resisted the limits of the dominant medical paradigms (homeopathy provides a prime example) as well as others that have recently begun to be tolerated as alternative and complementary medicines.[41] Foucault characterized these "disqualified" knowledges as representing "what people know . . . a particular knowledge that is local, regional, or differential, incapable of unanimity which derives its power solely from the fact that it is different from all the knowledges surrounding it . . . the non-commonsensical knowledges that people have, and which have in a way been left to lie fallow, or even kept in the margins."[42] *On Learning to Heal* seeks to recover and to value some of these excluded possibilities that lie fallow all around us in order to remind us that healing happens, and that while medicine might know some ways to enhance and augment this process, it does not have a monopoly on them. Moreover, it argues that until medicine appreciates healing as a vital tendency that lives in all of us, we might need not only to become aware of but also to learn to appreciate what medicine doesn't and probably can't know.

## ONE

## Healing Tendencies

Of all the objects treated by medical thought, healing is the one that doctors have considered least often.—GEORGES CANGUILHEM, "Une pédagogie de guérison" (1978)

Sometimes shit happens that completely changes the way we live. In my case, I had a radical healing experience. Nothing in my life had prepared me for this event, so it completely rocked my world. Of course, that's what *radical* means: it shakes you to the root. I was twenty-three at the time and had been living with acute Crohn's disease since I was thirteen. If you know anything about Crohn's— perhaps from the ads that now appear on TV for Remicade and Humira—you might know that it's an inflammatory autoimmune disease that can affect the entire gut from the mouth to the anus, causing diarrhea, intestinal pain, fistulas, and a panoply of other unpleasantness. When it first flared up in me, the inflammation involved the entire lining of my small bowel, so technically it was also regional enteritis (a term not much used anymore). *Flaring* is the official idiom to describe acute episodes of Crohn's, and it's an acutely apt indication of how your anus feels when it occurs. As a result of these fecal fireworks, I ended up being more or less—mostly more—incontinent throughout adolescence and young adulthood, which, needless to say, is a shitty way to grow up (pun definitely intended). Then, after enduring a decade-long deluge of diarrhea, I began to lose my shit entirely.

Just as I embarked on my PhD in modern thought at Stanford, my sphincters flailed against the relentless fecal fluids. In an (ultimately vain) attempt to stanch the flow, my doctors ordered ever-increasing doses of prednisone, then the go-to immunosuppressing corticosteroid, still used to tame all sorts of acute inflammations, from bad cases of poison ivy to lethal brain tumors. Because this was years before the current so-called biologic treatments like Remicade and Humira existed, prednisone was the most powerful prescription available, and I had been ingesting it in sometimes larger, sometimes smaller daily doses since my original diagnosis a decade earlier, albeit with decidedly mixed results. Yet despite the all-out pharmacological assault, the shitstorm did not let up, nor did the increasing torrent of side effects that the prednisone provoked. Then, in the spring of my second year at Stanford, on a visit to my parents, my intestines shut down completely. The ensuing intestinal obstruction (one of the other distinctive delights of Crohn's) landed me in a crappy doctors' hospital near where they lived. By sheer bad luck, this small medical center did not have a gastroenterologist on staff, so no one noticed that my small bowel had perforated. Instead, they pumped me full of painkillers, and once the blockage "resolved itself" (as they said), they released me. This turned out to be a fateful—and in fact almost fatal—flaw.

Once the contents of your gut break loose from their container, they're free to flourish in the warm, moist environs of your abdominal cavity, which can act like a high-end spa for bacteria. In my case, they started growing into colonies along the outside of my intestinal wall next to a major blood vessel, as well as migrating to my liver, where they multiplied with abandon—though this was only ascertained a few months later, after the emergency surgery that saved my life. For a month or so after the obstruction, nothing seemed much different than before. A lot of shit, all the time. However, once the abscesses grew large enough, they started to make themselves known in rather untoward ways.

One night while I was at the movies, envying the characters inhabiting the disembodied cyber world of Disney's *Tron* (who as two-dimensional characters had no guts to go awry), an abscess on my intestine burst. Since I (incorrectly) identified the sudden buildup of pressure as my old friend explosive diarrhea, I rushed home, clamping down on my by-then-considerably-developed sphincters with my by-then-considerably-developed might, reaching the toilet just as blood began gushing out my ass. When my housemates found me passed out in a bloody pool on the bathroom floor, they called an ambulance, which whisked me to Stanford University Hospital.

One of the world's foremost biomedical institutions, Stanford was, needless to say, nothing like the local hospital where my perforated bowel had gone undetected. They did every kind of test available and then some, yet they couldn't determine the cause of the bleeding and released me to the care of my gastroenterologist. More testing and even more prednisone ensued, still with no conclusive results. Then another major bleeding episode landed me back in the hospital. This time I started spiking high fevers at regular eighteen-hour intervals. The clockwork-like repetition clued my doctors in to the fact that I had some kind of serious infection, but who knew what kind or where? Again, they admitted me for even more tests. This time it would be several months before I emerged.

I can't remember why I ended up in a private room in the Hoover Pavilion, the posh part of the hospital—perhaps because it was the beginning of the AIDS epidemic, and I was a young gay man with an undiagnosed life-threatening infection living in the San Francisco Bay area. More tests, more fevers, more bleeding ensued. It was decided that I needed exploratory surgery, probably to remove a large part of my small intestine. Due to bad timing, however, before that could happen I had one final, massive bleed-out in the middle of the night. This time the bleeding would not stop. The more blood they pumped into me, the more it streamed out my anus. I could tell it was really bad, not only because my room was filled with doctors and nurses frantically trying to stabilize my blood pressure and get me to emergency surgery before I died but also because I was hovering above myself looking down on all this chaos with an incredibly calm detachment. Since I wasn't normally a super-calm person, I guessed that something unusual must be going on. Everything seemed very, very far away, even though I was right there watching it all. When they finally got me stable enough to race me to the operating room, I remember flying down the hallways—literally—watching myself on the gurney as nurses ran next to me, carrying the bags of blood and saline that adorned my appendages. The next thing I knew, I woke up in great pain in the ICU with tubes protruding from every available orifice.

That's when the healing began. It happened in a flash. A boy with whom I was madly but unrequitedly in love appeared at the door of my room, and I held out my IV-studded hand. When he took it, a surge of light went through me, and something changed. Though I had no idea at the time, I now mark that as the moment that life returned me to the world. The days in the ICU remain a haze—massive amounts of painkillers and antibiotics will do that to you. I learned that I'd had a small bowel resection, as predicted, and that they'd also discovered that my liver was filled with abscesses, which they'd drained.

I would now have to be on IV antibiotics until all signs of infection receded, and I would also have to be abruptly weaned off the cortisone steroids I'd been consuming in mass quantities for over ten years, because they impeded tissue healing. Not a great combination under the best of circumstances, especially not for someone as sick as me. After a week on the postsurgical ward, they returned me to my private room in the Hoover, so they could monitor me as the toxic drugs dripped into my veins and I simultaneously began steroid withdrawal. They would pump me full of one powerful antibiotic until I became allergic to it, and then they would switch to another and then another and then another. (I'm now allergic to lots of antibiotics.) Drop by toxic drop, the antibiotics poisoned the pastures, which is to say my viscera, where the errant bacteria thrived. Then, in the midst of this massive biochemical barrage, things got really interesting. Lying on my hospital bed, plugged into my Sony Walkman and drugged to the gills, I began to go into trances.

Everything in my life up until then had taught me that nothing like this could ever happen. My father was a physical chemist and my mother a naive but heartfelt Marxist; both were cultural Jews, committed materialists, and ardent atheists. My mother even belonged to the American Atheists organization founded by Madalyn Murray O'Hair (later kidnapped and gruesomely murdered by one of her former employees), so copies of *American Atheist* magazine could be found stacked on the corner of our dining room table. Nevertheless, despite my acquired atheistic affinities, the trances came upon me. At the time, I thought of them as pain management. With music streaming into my ears—it didn't matter whether it was Dire Straits, the Grateful Dead, or Yo-Yo Ma playing Bach's cello suites—I found I could enter into the spaces between the notes, where a peaceful realm filled with light opened out. Somehow (although I couldn't tell you how) I could take the light and mold it, wrapping it around the surgical wounds where my excised bowel and liver sought to refashion themselves. With that cushion of light between me and the pain, I would fall even deeper into the light-filled tranquility as everything else dropped away.

For a while this freaked my doctors and nurses out: they would come into my room and try to get my attention, but I'd be completely dead to the world. However, they soon learned that when they turned the music off, I'd quickly come out of it; after that, no one seemed to think that anything unusual was going on, including me. The trances became a regular part of my day, a relief from residual pain and encroaching boredom, as my body went about the work of repairing itself. I don't know what happened during these interludes. I had no grand plan; yet something apparently did. It seemed as if my body had a mind of its own. In the intervals where "I" receded into the music, the cells and molecules that constitute me tended toward my healing and toward healing me (whatever *me* now referred to). This healing tendency had nothing to do with my intention. I didn't even know that such a thing could happen, since no one ever seemed to have mentioned it to me before. It turned out my cells and molecules were way more intelligent than I was. They still are.

Because in those days insurance still reimbursed long hospitalizations, I remained in the Hoover Pavilion for another eight weeks. Friends visited; my mother sat by my bed reading her political tracts; I wandered the hallways pushing my IV pole and made friends with several others on my floor; we'd go up on the roof and get stoned. All in all, it was a peaceful time, especially compared to the Sturm und Drang that preceded it. Finally, it was decided that I was ready to leave the hospital and return to civilian life. As part of the transition, I had an exit interview with my surgeon. While I no longer remember his name, I do remember how handsome he was and that I'd developed a terrific crush on him. In our exit interview, he said something that completely changed my life. I've never forgotten his exact words: "You were the sickest person I've operated on in five years, who is still alive," he told me, "and I have no idea how you got better so quickly." His simple statement shocked me into a new reality.

On the one hand, it cut through the denial that I'd steadfastly maintained about just how sick I had been. Despite my out-of-body, near-death experience (which I didn't recognize as such at the time), I'd never really allowed myself to comprehend that I had been mortally ill. Instead, I'd told myself that this was just another phase of Crohn's—albeit more unpleasant and a little bit scarier than those that had gone before—and that I'd get through it as always. Although that did come to pass, it seems I'd been deluding myself about its likelihood. On the other hand, it also made me stop to actually consider: How had I gotten better so quickly? I'd been acutely and sometimes critically ill for the last ten years. Now I was supposedly getting "well"? After all the shit that had gone before, what had just happened? And why didn't my sexy surgeon know what had occurred? If he didn't, who did? More important, how had something unknown to this clearly accomplished, highly trained Stanford surgeon done me so much good?

Healing is not something you hear a lot about from most doctors. Disease is their bailiwick, and they're increasingly good at diagnosing and describing, if not always treating, it. Healing, however, doesn't take up as much space in their worldview. Today, if you look up *healing* on Medline, the US National Library of Medicine's comprehensive database, you will find only four categories: faith healing, fracture healing, mental healing, and wound healing. Not healing as a possibility, as a tendency, as a vital function, or as that upon which all of medicine's most prized bioscientific interventions depend. Yet for most of Western history, if not most of human history, healing was considered a vital function. In the Galenic/Hippocratic tradition that prevailed from antiquity until the middle of the nineteenth century, it was known in the same way that Hildegard of Bingen knew it, as the *vis medicatrix naturae*: the healing power of nature.[1] Although young doctors still faithfully intone the Hippocratic oath as part of their initiation rituals, the healing presumption from which it derived has long since been abandoned as the essential ethos of their training.

While many of us now suppose that medicine aspires to "cure" us—hence all the slogans and ribbons devoted to "cures" (e.g., the cure for cancer, the cure for AIDS, the cure for diabetes, the cure for MS)—cure is more or less a mythic phenomenon. It's aspirational, not empirical. Mostly, medicine manages disease—especially those diseases, such as Crohn's, that are deemed chronic. Healing desires something else. Healing does not ask: How can I get rid of this disease? Or, if not get rid of it, at least how can I "control" it? Rather, healing wonders: What can I learn from this disruptive-yet-vital experience? Can I develop and grow from this event—as Hildegard's invocation of *viriditas* suggests? Can I become myself more intensely and gracefully through this process, and if so, how? Can I learn to live otherwise? To live better? Neither cure nor management, healing gestures toward a different way of living with illness, or indeed of valuing it as a mode and means of living, one that medicine as we know it seems to have neglected, or perhaps forgotten.

I have no memory that any of my many doctors ever mentioned the possibility of healing. If they did, clearly I did not think it applied to me. Instead, I believed that the best I could hope for was to cope with my illness by faithfully complying with their recommendations and consuming the toxic drugs they prescribed. Alas, their bitter little pills never quite worked as promised, so shit was always happening, and I was constantly racing to find a convenient toilet before it happened in my pants. At the time, I imagined that this would be my lot for life—even as I had a vague sense, which I tried very hard to repress, that Crohn's might also impinge on my longevity.

From my current perspective, the initial diagnosis, along with its accompanying intimations of mortality and its pharmaceutically induced, hormonal override (my doctors explained how prednisone works by saying, "Prednisone overrides your adrenal glands"), effectively replaced the bar-mitzvah-that-I-never-had as a rite of passage into manhood—such as it was. Of course, that's not how I saw it then. Instead, because I was a teenage boy, I didn't give, or tried not to give, any of it too much thought and attempted to live what I now refer to as my "adolescence on steroids" as normally as a chronically ill, proto-queer, commie Jewish kid, living in a predominantly Catholic and conservative small town in semirural America in the early 1970s, could (all the while carrying several changes of underwear with me "just in case"). The notion that I might heal with Crohn's—if not *from* it—that I might live a different relation to it *and to myself* than the one my doctors described, never occurred to me. As dependent as I felt on their care, I took their words as truth; sadly, healing was no longer one of them. That turned out to be a decisive deficiency in vocabulary, since it neglected a very powerful resource to which I might have had access—if I'd had any inkling that it mattered. Until you can imagine a possibility, you cannot begin to cultivate it.

Of course, some doctors (like Victoria Sweet) do care about healing and try to encourage it. Alas, they're an underrepresented minority in this age of high-tech, evidence-based, computer-mediated, profit-driven health care, especially as it is underwritten (in all senses) by the insurance industry. So, despite some wonderful exceptions, from whom I've learned a lot and about whom I write in later chapters, it troubles me that the preponderance of medical practitioners in the United States have been taught to know so little about healing even though it is one of our most vital tendencies. To me this seems a crazy way to run a health care system, which in turn raises a few key questions: How and why did medicine, and especially medical training, forget that healing matters? What events helped refigure the medical imagination such that healing got demoted to a bit player, whereas for a long time it had been the star of the show? In other words, why does healing no longer take pride of place within medical discourse and education? After all, when biologists discuss the origins of life, they remind us that the basic functions that all organisms have performed since the first cell sprang into life include localizing themselves in space, reproducing themselves across time, taking in nutrients, expelling toxins, *and repairing themselves*. Without these essential abilities, nothing remains alive for long.

In part, the limit to what medicine knows about healing occurred because it began to assume that medicine should act more like a science than an art. Although, strictly speaking, medicine itself is not a science, contemporary medicine relies on the evidence produced by bioscience to inform its ways of thinking. According to current bioscientific understanding, it should be possible to explain all our vital functions in terms of the fundamental properties common to all matter. This perspective, known as biochemical reductionism, has motivated scientifically inclined medicine for the last 150 years or so. It presumes that while living organisms might incorporate a peculiar if not unique arrangement of molecules, atoms, subatomic particles, and quantum vibrational fields, in principle they manifest nothing that the inanimate world doesn't as well. Needless to say, biochemical reductionism has catalyzed many amazing therapeutic advances, upon which those of us who have access to them, and who can afford to pay for them, rely. Because I would be dead without them, I am happy to serve as a poster child for their powers. Nevertheless, there may be something more to life—and to healing—than the reductionist position admits, a certain *je ne sais quoi* that may in fact help explain why my surgeon didn't know how, or why, I had gotten better so quickly.

Those of us who admit such nonreducible possibilities often get called vitalists. (Vitalism has taken many forms but basically refers to any perspective which holds that the activities of living organisms cannot be entirely accounted for in the same way that physical processes can.[2]) In bioscientific circles, this is a bit like calling someone a flat-earther.[3] Before my radical healing, I was a resolute reductionist, scoffing at the very idea of vitalism, associating it with the capitalist metaphysics that my mother regularly reviled as "the opiate of the masses." Loyal to my family's naive communist-scientific dogma, I believed that matter was all that mattered. After surviving my sojourn in the Hoover Pavilion, however, it began to dawn on me that my commitment to my parents' materialisms may have caused me to miss out on something vital, and that vital something—which may or may not have been entirely biochemical—may have been what kept me alive. In the wake of the psychic whiplash induced by my roller-coaster ride from deathly illness to the walking well, I gradually began to consider that not everything that matters can be a priori reduced to matter.

In order to grasp the impact of reductionist methods on Western medicine, it helps to have a bit of the backstory: two centuries before reductionism became biochemical, it started out as mechanical. Mechanism entered Western natural philosophy in the sixteenth and seventeenth centuries in part as a way of demystifying the world imagined by Renaissance thinkers like Marsilio Ficino, Paracelsus, and Giordano Bruno, who "viewed the material world, and indeed matter itself, as a locus of subtle powers and immanent forces, a dynamic network of invisible sympathies and antipathies."[4] Mechanism promised to tame the potential wildness and unpredictability of the matter that confronted these Renaissance philosophers and alchemists (who were often both at the same time) and instead proposed to render it tractable to empirical investigation. Reducing matter to an inanimate substrate, rather than a lively locus of creative activity, mechanism made matter (theoretically) subject to human mastery.

Mechanical reductionism is often credited with helping to accelerate the dissolving dominance of Galenic/Aristotelian models in Western medical thought, and hence it played a prominent role in writing the *vis medicatrix naturae* out of the medical imagination. The history of this reductionism often names René Descartes as one of its founding figures (along with his contemporaries and adversaries Marin Mersenne and Pierre Gassendi). In the mid-seventeenth century, in addition to asserting "I think, therefore I am," Descartes also claimed that living bodies, human as well as animal, could and should be understood as incorporating the cumulative effects of mechanical causes. He based this supposition on the prior assumption that bodies—whether living or not—consisted of spatially delimited or "extended" inert substance, the *res extensa*, governed by laws of motion that were themselves instituted and enforced by God. (The God part would eventually fall away over the course of the next century or so, although not without considerable resistance.) As material bodies, Descartes presumed, living organisms were composed of parts that were also extended matter and for all (his) intents and purposes functioned as animated machines. As he framed it in his *Meditations on First Philosophy*: "I might consider the body of a man as a kind of machine equipped with and made up of bones, nerves, muscles, veins, blood, and skin."[5]

Descartes's mechanism supposed that all of an organism's operations could be accounted for in terms of determinate, if not determinable, relations between bodily parts and their law-like interactions. This mechanist matrix reverberated with such famous seventeenth-century analogies as these: the heart acts like a pump, the lungs like a bellows, the kidneys as a filter, God as a divine watchmaker, and so on.[6] However, despite mechanism's metastatic metaphors—its "going viral," as we might say today—it was not clear from Descartes's explanation how a living organism could manifest vital functions not anticipated by the causal principles underlying the universe as a whole, nor why animated machines were built in the ways they were in the first place. (God stood in for these reasons.) Nevertheless, despite these limitations, mechanical physiology, or mechanism as applied to living human organisms, persisted; indeed, it still persists, albeit in updated modes, often referred to in the contemporary philosophy of biology as "the new mechanism."[7]

In the mid-nineteenth century, two hundred years after mechanism first began to matter, mechanical physiology got a significant upgrade to what we might call "biochemical mechanism," or Mechanism 2.0, when the experimental physiologist Claude Bernard convinced his contemporaries that in order to go on living, an organism must maintain an internal biochemical balance. (Bernard's insight got rebranded as "homeostasis" in the twentieth century.[8]) In his seminal book *Introduction à l'étude de médecine expérimentale* (1865), Bernard argued that what he dubbed the *milieu intérieur*—a somewhat oxymoronic concept, since it can mean something like "inner surroundings"—constituted the "real theater of life."[9] While the organism obviously lived in the world, which Bernard denominated the *milieu extérieur*, this exterior world only mattered to it, according to Bernard, insofar as it manifested an inner presence by setting the stage for the biochemical drama that the organism's vital processes enacted. Bernard thereby explicitly bracketed the organism's vital context in order to constitute it as a quasi-closed system for the purposes of scientific experimentation, since open systems resist easy biochemical and biophysical reduction.

However, in so doing—and in order to do so—he also "derealized" the *milieu extérieur* as irrelevant to the vital theater that reductionist science examined in the lab. Thus, for Bernard and those who followed him, the *milieu intérieur* constituted the vital context in which nature's scripts came to life. (This "scripting" of biomedical interventions according to descriptions, prescriptions, inscriptions, and transcriptions gets taken up in chapter 2.[10]) The significance of Bernard's concept not only continues to consecrate laboratory-based bioscientific experimentation today, as well as most current clinical practice, but it also represents a definitive break with the Hippocratic/Galenic tradition that had prevailed in the West for the preceding two thousand years. As Canguilhem describes it, Bernard's intervention constituted not just a "historical rupture which inaugurates modern medicine" but also "a declaration of war on Hippocratic medicine."[11] This bellicose orientation has characterized medicine's preferred methods ever since.

The earlier paradigm, from which the *vis medicatrix naturae* derived and which Bernard's intervention rendered increasingly obsolete, based its approach on the idea that living bodies are composed of humors, elements, and cardinal qualities. It supposed that healthy bodies balance these elemental requirements and that, conversely, illnesses result from imbalances among them. Such "bad mixtures" (*dyskrasia*) could arise within the organism, between the organism and its environment, or both. Consequently, the physician's responsibility was to recognize such imbalances and help rectify them through a combination of regimen (regulating food, drink, exercise, rest, habitat, etc.), pharmacopoeia (largely plant and mineral based), and surgery (only if absolutely necessary). These therapeutic interventions presumed that with the right support and encouragement, an organism would tend to reestablish its own natural humoral harmony. However, after Bernard's experimental intervention, two thousand years of humoral thinking quickly fell from grace.[12] Instead of invoking the *vis medicatrix naturae*, Bernard introduced the now-familiar vocabulary of warfare into medicine. Describing his belief that medical therapies should act as "arms" and "weapons" (which at the time was an entirely unrealized, aspirational agenda), he planted the notion that an organism's struggles with disease are primarily defensive, rather than reparative or restorative. Until then, no one thought that healing was primarily defensive, or that defense was healing—but that was about to change.

In the wake of Bernard's biochemical split, vitalism in medicine took a massive hit. Biochemical reductionism increasingly seemed able to provide answers to persistent problems for which vitalists could offer no real redress. The late nineteenth century witnessed the emergence of the new sciences of bacteriology and immunology, which sought to explain, if not ameliorate, the causes of infectious diseases, especially epidemic ones. It also beheld the introduction of the first attenuated vaccines that were effective against them.[13] (Chapter 3 explains in detail how these new sciences shaped scientific medical education at the beginning of the twentieth century.) Because they promised to act preemptively on individuals in order to protect populations, these new public health technologies certainly seemed miraculous. Whereas earlier in the century, the best hope against mass infection had rested on rather tenuous quarantines and *cordons sanitaires*, which attempted to restrict people's movements into or out of distinct geographical regions (often by military means), the new protocols offered effective prophylaxis against large-scale pathogenic "attack." Hence, the new vaccines introduced the possibility of not only managing epidemic morbidity and mortality but also assuaging the perturbing political and economic consequences that epidemics inevitably entailed as well.

At the same time, and as a result, these vaccines were also the first profitable products of the world's first biotech enterprise, the Pasteur Institute (partly in support of European colonial expansion in Africa, Asia, and Latin America). Thus, they demonstrated for the first time that health care could make a significant contribution to both capitalism and imperialism.[14] Soon thereafter, bioscientists began introducing chemical compounds—often the dyes used to stain bacteria to render them visible under a microscope—as antimicrobial chemotherapies that would "fight disease," anticipating the advent of the antibiotics that have inundated us since the middle of the twentieth century. In so doing, they also catalyzed the pharmaceutical industry that has so successfully capitalized upon them. Yet, as my surgeon's remarks intimated, despite these manifest successes, there remained, and still remains, much about life that biochemical reductionism does not and cannot explain. Indeed, it may be the case that although reductionism has much to offer us both conceptually and practically, it is not all that we often suppose.

$$\maltese$$

This is not a new idea. In fact, at the very moment that late nineteenth and early twentieth-century bioscientific advances were transforming not only what medicine could do but also what it actually was, the French philosopher Henri Bergson suggested that rather than simply revel in the knowledge that bioscientific reductionism brought, we might at least acknowledge that we can't know everything—if only so that our (supposed) knowingness doesn't get in the way of learning, or perhaps creating, something new. Bergson's critiques of mechanism and determinism, the principles that buttress biochemical reductionism, appeared in his book *Creative Evolution* (1907), one of the main texts for which he was awarded the Nobel Prize in Literature in 1927. According to Bergson, determinate knowledge—of which modern science represents the pinnacle—constitutes one of the ways that human life has evolved in order to extend itself in time and space. He held that in evolutionary terms, determinate knowledge of material phenomena, derived by breaking down dynamic processes into separate moments or calculable states, definitely enhances the ways humans act in and on the world. It thereby helps us survive, if not thrive, as living organisms. Yet he argued that despite its obvious value in helping us negotiate our ways through the material world and its usefulness in enhancing our lives, determinism alone can't encompass the ongoing innovations of life—including human life. This creative capacity seemed to him an essential if undervalued aspect of life as we know it.[15]

In other words, while Bergson did not reject the determinism that allows us to know life analytically or scientifically, he nevertheless believed that such knowledge in itself cannot encompass all that living entails, and especially not human living. Instead, he argued that since we are living beings ourselves, we can never separate ourselves from life enough to know it "objectively" (as long as we remain alive). Thus, he proposed, we also need to cultivate what he called "intuition" in order to apprehend and appreciate "the inwardness of life."[16] Intuition for Bergson represents a sense of life that arises from within the ongoing duration of living, from within life processes. As such, it resists the parsing of our vital nature into static moments for the purposes of scientific analysis because these processes are not just states strung together one after another, just as a line is not a string of points.[17] Only by cultivating our capacity to immerse ourselves in the "river of time" and by developing the vital ability to go with the temporal flow, Bergson insisted, can we begin to grasp valuable aspects of our existence that will always elude us if we merely try to snag them from the river's tangled banks.[18]

In the era before genetics, half a century before the discovery of DNA (which for a time seemed to confirm reductionism and therefore rendered Bergson's insights too simple to be of much further scientific interest), Bergson characterized the impetus for intuition, and indeed for all life, in terms of what he called the *élan vital*. For Bergson, the *élan vital* impels and propels life into inanimate matter. Incorporating this original impulse (*élan original*), life manifests "a certain contingency entering into the world—that is to say a certain quantity of possible action."[19] In fact, Bergson states that it is the "role of life . . . to insert some indetermination into matter";[20] or, to put it slightly differently, life makes matter(s) more complicated. Needless to say, contingency and indetermination do not subscribe to determinism's distinctive ways of thinking about change. If something is determined, there is no contingency or indetermination, and vice versa. For Bergson, the *élan vital* gestured toward the paradoxical possibility that a contingent indetermination, impelled by a movement within matter, introduces new degrees of change (which he thought might be another name for creativity). Moreover, it names a tendency of matter that enables it to stretch itself toward new possibilities, to manifest new forms of freedom, by inventing new forms of life.

Reductionist critics have dismissed the *élan vital* as a metaphysical rather than physical concept, accusing Bergson of being a vitalist in order to disqualify his perspective as insufficiently objective or scientific—and hence, by implication, invalid. Yet this is not entirely what Bergson had in mind. In fact, Bergson did not see himself as a vitalist at all and instead regarded unreflective vitalism as simply another kind of determinism. Nevertheless, he also maintained that vitalism offered a helpful corrective to the deterministic prejudices of reductionism: "the vital principle may indeed not explain much," he wrote, "but it is at least a sort of label affixed to our ignorance, to remind us of it occasionally."[21]

Bergson's ironically understated reminder remains salient. Certainly, the law of unintended consequences applies as much to bioscience as to any other domain. For example, the invention of antibiotics (to which I and many, many others owe our lives) has also led to their overuse by both medicine and agribusiness, resulting in the increasing proliferation of antibiotic-resistant bacteria for which we currently have no effective treatments. Or, to invoke another ironic twist of fate, the medical triumph that resulted in the elimination of naturally occurring smallpox has transformed what was once an endemic, although sometimes epidemic, viral disease into one of the most powerful bioweapons in existence. But even though they reveal the limits of bioscientific knowledge to predict its own effects, these examples still fail to capture the full significance of Bergson's admonition.

When Bergson asks us to remember our ignorance, he does not imagine that ignorance will someday be replaced by—or, indeed, reduced by—scientific knowledge. Rather, he challenges us to recognize that as living beings we are not only constitutively more complicated than we know but perhaps more complicated than we can ever know: "Nature is what it is, and as our intelligence, which is a part of it, is less vast than nature, it is doubtful whether any of our present ideas is large enough to embrace it. . . . Let us not shrink reality to the measure of our ideas."[22] Simply put: knowledge does not exhaust our resources for living, let alone living well, or maybe even living better. In this regard, our knowledge about living is paradoxical, for knowing only develops within life (human life, if not other life forms) as a way of extending and enhancing it. So how could this part of life ever come to know everything about the vital terrain from which it arises, on which it depends, to which it returns, and which always extends beyond it in both time and space?

I didn't know anything about Bergson when the sudden experience of healing overtook me. Yet a few decades later, when I got around to reading *Creative Evolution*, it immediately helped me make sense of it. Until then, I'd never thought of ignorance as an asset—especially not in relation to illness. When you're very sick, you really want someone to know what's going on, and, even more, you hope that what that someone knows can help you go on living. Turns out that's a lot to ask. Yet many of us do it every day, usually without thinking. We take pills; we get surgeries; we endure chemo; we schedule checkups—always desiring that what our physicians know might relieve our suffering, if not save our lives. Behind our doctors, we also implicitly trust the bioscientists who augment the knowledge base on which they (and hence we) depend. And behind these bioscientists, we rely on the biomedical institutions and biotech corporations that employ them to decide which knowledge will generate enough profit to warrant developing. Medicine invests in knowing, and we invest in that investment, financially as well as psychically, with our bodies, our minds, and our wallets.

To invoke an idiom made famous by the French psychoanalyst Jacques Lacan, who also trained as a doctor, we approach a physician as a *sujet supposé savoir*, as a "subject who is supposed to know."[23] However, in doing so we might fail to notice that the word *supposed* points in two directions here: toward us, it underscores our desire, our supposition, about what a doctor can do for us; toward the doctors, it emphasizes that knowing is supposed to be—that is, should be—their stock in trade. This is not entirely surprising, since medicine has been a knowledge enterprise from the very outset. What distinguished a physician like Hippocrates from a temple healer, a prophet, an herbalist, a midwife, or any other contemporary practitioner was the faith that knowledge alone would provide the best therapy. (The Greeks invented the word *iatrike* in the fifth century BCE to name this new knowing commitment.) That's why diagnosis has always served as medicine's trademark: in Greek, it literally means "by way of knowledge" (*dia + gnosis*).

Don't get me wrong: I'm all for knowledge. As my friends will tell you, if you haven't already guessed, I can be an annoying know-it-all. Nevertheless, when I belatedly came upon Bergson's ironic affirmation of the vital principle as "a sort of label affixed to our ignorance, to remind us of it occasionally," I wondered if this idea might also helpfully apply to healing as well. Perhaps, I thought, contemporary medicine's ignorance of healing results from its overinvestment in knowing, from asking too much of it. Maybe acknowledging our irreducible ignorance—as Atlan proposed—as well as our potential for knowledge could give us access to resources that we have undervalued. To put this another way: What if ignorance doesn't simply name that which knowledge must reduce or overcome, if not eliminate? What if it also marks an opening or a gap in our understanding of the world that can turn us toward something that exceeds our grasp yet which nevertheless also invites it? "Not knowing," which is what *ignorance* (from the same Greek root as *diagnosis*) means etymologically, does not necessarily name a pure negativity, an absence, a void, or an emptiness where something ought to be. It can also allude to an attitude that attends to more-than-knowing, other-than-knowing, not-*just*-knowing.

In Zen Buddhism, for example, not-knowing is sometimes called "beginner's mind" (*shoshin*) and refers to an unassuming attitude of curiosity that lacks preconceptions and thereby opens us to new, heretofore unknown, possibilities.[24] Beginner's mind indicates that if properly appreciated, ignorance might encourage us to turn our attention toward that which remains unknown or unknowable, toward that which lies beyond the bounds of our knowing's ambitions. Perhaps by acknowledging our ignorance, then, we could even take more advantage of it. Embracing healing as a vital aspect of our inevitable ignorance, as a way of naming that which cannot be reduced to the movements of matter alone, does not require that we forego medicine's knowing ways. Rather, it might only require that we forego the arrogance and hubris that assume we must know, or even that we can know, the outcomes of all our therapeutic adventures in advance.

Personally, I don't know what healing is, only what it can do, or at least what it has done for me. Although I certainly experienced it, I still don't know how it happened; hence, I wouldn't want to swear to its truth. For years I downplayed my healing process and didn't discuss it because I couldn't prove it was true. (Of course, we now live in what many deem a "post-truth" era, so maybe this no longer really matters.) Yet in medical contexts, especially given prevailing evidence-based orientations, the quest for truth still provides the gold standard for sorting among therapeutic options. That's why clinical trials have taken on such importance and why they have spawned an international industry that profits by conducting them around the globe.[25] Because clinical trials seem to enact and therefore incorporate the scientific method, they both create and legitimate the notion that there exists a measurable correspondence between a treatment and its therapeutic outcomes. They do this by repeatedly administering the treatment being tested to a representative population of potential users. (We return to the assumptions that underwrite this bio-logic of testing in chapter 3.)

Needless to say, such treatments must also be potentially profitable commodities, or no one would bother to pay for the trials.[26] These trials then produce data that are subjected to complex statistical assessments. These analytic interpretations then turn into reams of documents that are reviewed by state-endorsed entities, which in turn decide whether the treatments can be legally prescribed—and hence profited from by both patients and pharmaceutical corporations. Trials translate the repetition of treatments into data by establishing a numerical consistency that equalizes each instance of the treatment to every other instance. These repetitions substantiate the conclusions drawn from the data as if each instance of treatment in the trial was the same and therefore interchangeable, implying that every trial subject is interchangeable as well. Ever since Descartes wrote his *Discourse on Method* (1637), such "objective" repeatability has served as the benchmark for establishing scientific truth. If the preponderance of repetitions produces enough positive therapeutic results, this repeatability validates a treatment's effectiveness.

In relation to this gold standard (as double-blind clinical trials are called in medical discourse), my radical experience of healing appears merely anecdotal. Its nonrepeatable nature undermines its potential validity, if not its significance. Indeed, I'm happy that (so far) it has remained a once-in-a-lifetime experience, which is why I keep trying to learn what it still has to teach me so as not to repeat it. Yet even though I cannot say for certain what happened, or how it happened, or why it happened, that doesn't mean it didn't happen. Biomedically speaking, *certainty* refers to having a high confidence in the statistical likelihood of repeatability (where this confidence is calculated in comparison to a placebo). Such statistics presume predictable probabilities, which are implicitly considered to be calculable, and therefore (at least in theory) both knowable and enumerable. For example, when oncologists are asked to provide prognoses—often in response to a question like, "Doc, how much time do I have?"—they prefer to specify survival rates as probabilities or chances instead of presenting individualized time frames. Conversely, they are often troubled at doing so because they recognize the impossibility of accounting for any specific case in such statistical terms.

*Probability* only came to refer to the measurable likelihood of an occurrence during the eighteenth century, when the calculus of probabilities was first invented.[27] Thereafter, probabilities started to be calculated in terms of ratios (e.g., "she has a three-in-ten chance of surviving the operation at her age") as a way of referring to what previously would have simply appeared uncertain. Probability seeks to contain uncertainty by converting its troubling ambiguities into numbers, thereby giving it the veneer of knowability and predictability.[28] And since medicine trades in the therapeutic power of knowledge, it prefers to think in terms of probabilities rather than possibilities. However, the probable is not the same as the possible, because probability only pertains to phenomena whose regularities we can calculate. Yet improbable things happen all the time—including healing—even if we can't count (on) them.

When probability begins to underwrite the basic bio-logic of biomedicine, the value of improbable experiences, even those in which we might have great confidence (albeit without statistical confirmation) diminishes. This explains why, in the medical archive, instances of radical healing, for example spontaneous remission from cancer, though well documented, get minimized as merely anecdotal.[29] Nevertheless, to those of us who have lived through them, such results are as real as any biomedically induced remission—even if neither we nor our doctors know why or how they occurred. The fact is: the resources that knowledge affords us, as powerful as they can be, may not entirely capture the healing events we experience. Thus, while I may not be able to repeat it, I am happy to affix the name *healing* to my ignorance of what happened to me, and of what I have witnessed happen to others, in order to remind myself of it from time to time. Or, to embrace ignorance even more enthusiastically, let me proclaim: all I know is that healing happened to me in a very radical and improbable way, and I'm very, very glad that it did. Once I began to recognize this unknown experience for what it was, to acknowledge it, to pay attention to it, and to begin to appreciate and cultivate it in myself, I began to be able to recognize, acknowledge, attend to, appreciate, and help cultivate it in others.

Needless to say, despite my professed ignorance, I do have a few thoughts about healing, since I have obviously benefited from the experience. One of these thoughts concerns what we mean by *experience* per se. How does experience inform us? What difference does experience make to how we live our lives? And why do experiences of illness and healing often remain so remarkably vivid? One way to explain what experience has to offer is to consider it as a way life gives itself to being thought about by living beings (i.e., us) from within life. This insider understanding distinguishes experience from scientific knowledge, which tries to establish an external, aka "objective," vantage point from which to consider life without either the tint or the taint—take your pick—of subjectivity. Although *experience* and *experiment* share the same etymology, the latter has come to refer to the work that science performs in order to objectively validate knowledge, whereas the former seemingly slides toward subjective bias. The philosopher Thomas Nagel famously characterized scientific objectivity as a "view from nowhere," which of course could also mean a view from everywhere.[30]

Etymologically, *experience* comes from the Latin *experior* (meaning to try, to prove, to undertake, to attempt, to undergo, etc.), which in turn derives from a Greek root πειρα (to try, to attempt, to experience) that also resonates with another Greek word περάω (to pierce, to penetrate, to traverse, to pass through a space).[31] This chain of meanings links experience to life itself in the sense that Bergson underscores: "the living being is above all a thoroughfare, and . . . the essence of life is in the movement by which life is transmitted."[32] In other words, following Bergson, we might affirm that experiences underscore the vital ways life travels through our lives, urging us in new directions, opening us to new opportunities. Experience names the ways we are traversed, penetrated, pierced by forces we do not and cannot know but which nonetheless move us and move within us.

Illness is by definition an experience; until it catches our attention, it doesn't exist as such.[33] This doesn't mean precipitating conditions might not be unfolding in our lives before we cotton on to them: we might live in toxic environments, work at toxic jobs, engage in toxic relations, consume too many toxic substances. We might have genetic predispositions, acquired vulnerabilities, repetitive stresses and strains that wear away at our vitality. However, until their effects impinge on us and thereby attract our attention, their significance has not been suffi-ciently valued—or devalued—as illness. Because illness, unlike disease, names an experience, it does not succumb to medicine's taxonomies or histories. Ill-nesses do not partake of the generalities that define the parameters of disease diagnoses. Instead, they characterize the specificities that disrupt our usual going-on-living in untoward ways. Illnesses represent intervals during which our normal life patterns can no longer meaningfully support the values by which we seek to live.[34] Hence, while diseases may carve out subsets of popu-lations that can be statistically analyzed according to current epidemiological categories, for illnesses the motto remains: to each their own.[35]

Although there are competing theories of what a disease is, *disease* usu-ally refers to the way that medicine characterizes harmful transformations of matter and energy that affect or impede the normal functioning of an organism. Hence, diseases name what pathology defines as abnormal. As Canguilhem noted in his book *The Normal and the Pathological*: "What one finds in com-mon in the different meanings given to disease today and in the past is that they form a judgment of virtual value."[36] Yet while disease may reflect a value judgment about our vital conditions, it does not tell us how we make sense of, or live with, the transformations it describes—although the naming itself can affect our awareness in powerful ways. Consider the examples that Susan Son-tag made famous: the word *cancer*—which is not in fact a disease but a generic rubric that encompasses a cornucopia of cellular cacophonies—often deeply informs how people diagnosed with different metastatic conditions go on liv-ing their lives. The very name, Sontag argues, can unwittingly evoke a type of person who might be inclined to its metastases (e.g., having a "cancer person-ality").[37] Another rubric that attempted to encompass a plethora of possible symptomologies and to delimit a set of people who are at risk of manifesting it would be AIDS.[38] Crohn's disease is yet another. Illness, on the other hand, denotes an experience that disrupts our ability to function in the ways we con-sider valuable, if not desirable.

It's no coincidence that our word *value* comes from the Latin *valere*, which means, among other things, "to be healthy, strong, powerful, or well."[39] In other words, if health is valuable, illness conversely describes experiences that trouble our value(s). Illnesses call attention to themselves—and call our attention to them—by interfering with our lives in ways that make us "feel ill" or "feel sick" (which is why we don't usually say, "I feel diseased"). They may be connected to pathological manifestations that can be attributed to cellular and biochemi-cal changes, or not—as conditions like chronic fatigue syndrome, fibromyalgia, or chronic (or post-treatment) Lyme disease illustrate.[40] Hence, we refer to "mental illnesses" but not "mental diseases" because no robust biochemical explanations currently exist for them.[41] Although we often conflate the two, illness can tell us something about how we want to live, whereas disease tells us what a doctor decides is wrong. As the sociologist Arthur Frank noted in reflecting on his own experience of testicular cancer: "The common diagnostic categories into which medicine places its patients are relevant to disease, not illness. They are useful for treatment, but they get in the way of care."[42]

Unfortunately, I didn't even notice there was a difference between illness and disease until a number of years after my extended stay in the Hoover Pavilion, when the best doctor I ever met, who to my great good fortune happened to be both the world's expert on Crohn's disease and the father of a close friend, asked me a deceptively simple question: "So how has Crohn's affected your life?" It was only after his question landed that I realized, for the first time: Crohn's disease isn't my life. Until that moment it had never occurred to me that "my life" and "Crohn's" could be two separate things, no matter how profoundly the latter infected my experience of the former.

If there is one thing that my experience with Crohn's has definitely taught me, it is that healing is not a steady state. Like awareness, healing is intermittent at best. That's why I like to call it a tendency. *Tendency* derives from the Latin root *tendere*, meaning, among other things: to stretch, aim, strive, endeavor.[43] When we "tend" toward something, we can stretch toward it in a variety of ways (as the words at*ten*tion, in*ten*tion, re*ten*tion, pre*ten*sion, con*ten*tion, dis*ten*tion, etc., all derived from the same *ten-* root, indicate). Bergson argued that life consists of the disparate tendencies composed by the *élan vital*. To my mind, that's a pretty expansive way to think about it. However, we must keep in mind that *compose* does not necessarily mean "get along" or "agree"; tendencies also ignore, as well as oppose and contest, one another. Moreover, we don't contain all these tendencies in ourselves. Many of the most powerful tendencies that compose us, and of which we are composed, exist between us or among us—where *us* means not only all humans, or even all living beings, but also the biosphere, solar system, galaxy, and universe(s) as well. After all, gravity does tend to have a significant effect on our lives, as do technology and capitalism.

To elaborate on Bergson's image a bit: imagine that all of the tendencies that bear upon us, and that we bear and bear with, stream together, creating eddies and whirlpools within which, for shorter or longer periods of time, the effects that we think of as living appear. According to the second law of thermodynamics, no matter how long or short the intervals, these vital spirals of matter-energy must ultimately fold back onto themselves and into the general dissipating drift of the universe, also called entropy.[44] Each spiral's limited duration constitutes what we might call a life-time. Sometimes tendencies compose in ways that prevent such spirals from forming or that catalyze their collapse. Sometimes antientropic tendencies arise that sustain these spiral eddies in space-time, sometimes even enhancing their coherence, albeit only for a while. (Is this the place to reveal that my childhood nickname was Eddie?) To me, healing designates such an antientropic tendency, which we can (sometimes) cultivate and encourage, often with the help of others. Yet as a tendency it requires attention; it needs us to tend it as we tend to ourselves and others. Invoking healing explicitly seems to support this effort; appreciating it, if and when it happens, doesn't seem to hurt either. This book tends in both those directions.

However, before we extend this way of thinking—if not experiencing—much further, it's important to underscore that healing is not antideath because death is not the opposite of life.[45] Indeed, life as we know it, that is, human life, depends on death. Death is entailed in life. As embryos, the preponderance of our cells must die (via what is called apoptosis, or programmed cell death) in order for us to gestate properly. If not, we might either fail to be born or struggle with severe disabilities. Once out of the uterus, billions of our cells die daily, and if they don't die properly, we might manifest what we call cancer. Hence, not only is death not the opposite of life, it forms one of its conditions of possibility, one of its tendencies. Or, to put this another way, death is not the enemy of healing.

Unfortunately, ever since Claude Bernard began to describe medicine as an arsenal, the antideath ethos has been explicitly or implicitly enshrined in scientific medicine. In part, this death-defying drive derives from how dead bodies have functioned in the history of modern medicine. Since the end of the eighteenth century, when "opening up a few corpses" (the phrase belongs to Michel Foucault) established pathological anatomy as the basis for clinical medicine, the no-longer-living have played a special role in the medical imagination.[46] By correlating symptoms witnessed when patients were dying with lesions discovered during autopsies, medicine began to certify the consistent correlations between tissue damage and knowledge production that have bankrolled its business ever since. Needless to say, there's a lot to be learned about the effects of disease from a dead body; however, there's not much it can teach us about healing because healing is an attribute of the living. In fact, to learn about healing, you might need to be able to hold open the play between life and death as a productive as well as destructive tension.

Indeed, Canguilhem suggested that healing entails holding life and death together: "To learn to heal is to learn to experience [*connaitre*] the contradiction between today's hope and its failure in the end. Without saying no to today's hope. Is this intelligence or simplicity?"[47] The terms Canguilhem uses to frame his rhetorical question are telling: within life, the hope of going-on-living inevitably butts up against the fact of death on a daily basis. Healing expresses the friction that arises between these divergent tendencies, even as it yearns for more life. So why does Canguilhem ask if this is intelligence or simplicity? Why oppose the two? First of all: Why intelligence? *Intelligence* derives from a Latin preposition, *inter* (between, amid, among, in the midst of), and a complex Latin verb, *legere*. *Legere* can mean, among many other things, to gather, to collect, to glean, to choose, to read.[48] Intelligence thus suggests a kind of gathering, collecting, gleaning, choosing, or reading from in between—as in "reading between the lines." Intelligence discloses what is implicit in the complicated and makes it explicit. In other words, and quite literally, intelligence unfolds things—as the root *pli-* (meaning to fold), folded into im*pli*cate, com*pli*cate, and ex*pli*cate, indicates. Intelligence recognizes the entanglement of things, as well as their intrinsic non-self-evidence, and tries to glean new insights from the spaces or gaps tucked within what is already there. Gathering from the interstices, the intervals, that compose life's tendencies, intelligence bears upon that which is not yet known, that of which we have heretofore remained ignorant. (Bergson juxtaposes intelligence, instinct, and intuition as life's intertwined tendencies that sustain our survival in the material world.)

Simplicity, on the other hand, from the Latin *simplex*, refers to that which is unmixed, uncompounded, single, consisting of only one element; figuratively, it can indicate the moral qualities of frankness, directness, guilelessness, sincerity, honesty, candidness. Simplicity thus foregrounds unity, consistency, integrity, perhaps even identity. The simple has no in-between, no gaps, no fissures, no pleats, no wounds. It is what it is. When Canguilhem poses the rhetorical question of whether learning to heal is intelligence or simplicity, then, he is *not* asking: Is this smart? Is this stupid? Instead, he challenges us to recognize that the living contradictions that we are—and that we can only ever be—entail both our intelligence *and* our simplicity. We are many and yet we are one. We hope and our hope fails us. We are living and we are dying, always at the same time. Indeed, our living always tends toward one end: our death. Healing arises in the tension in between. It lives in us as that which sustains our lives, until it no longer does. That's why at best it's a tendency, not a fact, a force, a probability, a certainty, or an inevitability.

Healing tendencies require cultivation and care. Unlike cures, they demand careful curation, that is, not only an attentive selection and combination of therapeutic resources but also constant upkeep thereafter (that's why in museums curation involves maintenance and restoration as well as selection, framing, and arrangement). Cure relies on the fantasy that knowing correctly can produce a desired transformation in an undesirable situation by negating or eliminating that which is undesired, whether that be a disease (the cure for HIV/AIDS, the cure for cancer, the cure for MS, etc.), a socioeconomic condition (the cure for poverty, the cure for hunger, the cure for homelessness), or even a biopolitical challenge (the cure for income inequality, the cure for overpopulation, the cure for global warming). However, there are important differences between curing and caring: you can cure without caring, and you can care without curing—although these are certainly not mutually exclusive. Medical cures rely on knowledge as the basis for their therapeutic powers. With no disrespect to biomedicine, it might not yet know enough about how to care. Feminist scholars have long documented the gendered and racialized divisions of care within the medical-industrial complex. In hospitals, caring usually falls to nurses and nonmedical staff, while doctors claim a monopoly on knowledge. Of course, there are caring doctors too, but care is not their primary obligation.[49] Diagnosing and prescribing are. These critical practices constitute the physician's core concerns, and they have become increasingly intricate, along with the bioscience and biotechnologies that underwrite them. Spend any time in an ICU and you'll see what I mean. Yet healing resonates with care, and care amplifies healing; thus, when we care about healing, it matters.

*Care* is an interesting word. It comes from the Middle High German root *caren*, which means both trouble, grief, or sorrow, and the succoring thereof.[50] In his discussion of "the antithetical meaning of primal words," Freud compared this kind of folding together of contraries to what happens in our dreams, which are not governed by the laws of logic. While this may or may not be a reliable explanation for the opposing meanings that care carries, it does suggest why care might not lie at the heart of contemporary medicine's knowledge practices. Ever since Aristotle, who lived a hundred years after Hippocrates, the law of noncontradiction has governed the domain of knowledge production. Its corollary, the law of the excluded middle, also insists that for those who would know the truth, there is no middle way between what something is and what it is not (in direct contrast to Buddhism). Since the end of the eighteenth century, when medicine first began to aspire to scientific status, it has insisted on establishing a split among verifiable treatments, that is, those predicated on statistically revealed relations between causes and effects, and those which might produce effective results but whose cause-effect correlations cannot be reliably regulated. The former became the province of physicians; the latter, of quacks and charlatans and, more recently, practitioners of alternative medicine. (Chapter 3 addresses the genesis of this dominant bio-logic.)

While medicine's scientific precaution no doubt has good reason—in the double sense of logic and motivation—it may have thrown the baby out with the bathwater. Care can matter even when the causes of its mattering remain beyond our ken. Indeed, caring often entails both attending to suffering and attempting to relieve it, even when we cannot explain it. In this sense, caring can support and encourage healing by appreciating that it matters whether or not we know why or how. Therefore, learning to care might be contradictory, or at least it might require us to learn to live with ambiguities and contradictions, just like learning to heal. As Canguilhem suggests, it might involve both hope and the recognition that our hope won't keep us from dying sooner or later.

As you can probably tell by now, I am a fan of ambiguity and contradiction. Paradox, *c'est moi*. In part, that's an occupational hazard—I have a PhD in modern thought, and I am a professor at a major research university, so I've spent a lot of time dwelling in and on the tensions that knowing inevitably involves. But even as a child, this was both a blessing and a curse for me. People were always telling me I lived in my head, although I couldn't understand why that was a problem. And then as I got a bit older and became an incontinent teen, thinking seemed to offer a sanctuary from all that crazy shit my body was doing. If I could have become a perfect Cartesian subject simply by embracing the credo "I think, therefore I am," so that my being would only have involved thinking, I would gladly have signed up. Alas, my gut was my Achilles' heel. In a wonderful essay, "Mind and Its Relation to the Psyche-Soma," the English psychoanalyst Donald Winnicott helps us appreciate the paradoxical usefulness of this defensive aspect of thought. Mind, he suggests, emerges as a mental refuge for us as infants when our demands remain unsatisfied by those we require to sustain us. At this stage of our development, since we cannot fulfill our own needs for food, shelter, warmth, love, and so on by ourselves, we require others to fulfill them for us—otherwise we die. The downside of this is, whoever can fulfill our needs can also frustrate them. Winnicott argues that in early life, as a child reaches the limit of its ability to tolerate such frustration, it creates "mind" by hallucinating a satisfaction that it does not actually experience. This fantasizing helps it endure its frustration a bit longer, until an actual satisfaction occurs.

Mind thus serves as both a haven for and an escape from the vital demands of what Winnicott calls the "psyche-soma," our living-breathing-feeling-matter.

Unfortunately, if the child's environment obstructs its satisfaction too frequently or for too long, the child can begin to manifest a pathological proclivity toward mental activity as a substitute. Psychosomatic illnesses provided Winnicott with a prime example of this pathology. While somatic symptoms surface in such "psychic" conditions, often to the consternation of physicians who cannot identify their causes (and therefore cannot properly diagnose a disease), Winnicott argues that the "agent" of the illness can be attributed to a "dissociation in the patient," and it is the "persistence of this split . . . that constitutes the true illness."[51] Extrapolating from Winnicott's insight, we could hypothesize that all illness has some psychosomatic element insofar as illness (as distinct from disease) is by definition a frustrating experience. Be that as it may, even when it serves as a defense against frustration to a more or less pathological degree, mind can also reveal resources that allow us to innovate new, less pathological, ways of living. After all, that's why Winnicott wrote his essay in the first place—and why I am writing this book as well. If thinking can be a trap, it can also show us ways out, and sometimes it even helps to create them. Thinking thus provides a paradoxical possibility for dealing with all the shit that happens to us—including the actual shit that an illness like inflammatory bowel disease stirs up.

Unfortunately, the ways we think about medicine and disease—or the ways we learn to think about disease from medicine—do not usually figure prominently in how we engage our experiences of illness. Nevertheless, these forms of thought permeate us, not just conceptually but cellularly and biomolecularly. We incorporate them every time we take up the therapeutic interventions (e.g., vaccines, antibiotics, pharmaceuticals, surgeries) that biomedicine makes on our behalf. Medicine's ways of thinking matter—literally—insofar as their success depends on their capacity to inform and perhaps reform our tissues, cells, and molecules. As a consequence, biomedicine's ideas and technologies not only shape what we think is going on when we start feeling ill but also influence what we imagine can be done when we do. In our current context, that often means going to a doctor. In addition to everything else they might be able to do for us, our doctors often give us the terms with which— and within which—we grapple with illness. That includes a diagnosis, which, if nothing else, can give us the feeling that what we're experiencing can be known. When our doctors don't know what's wrong with us, we know we're probably in deep shit.

However, medicine's ways of thinking about disease do not exhaust the phenomena that illnesses manifest. Indeed, sometimes they constrain our abilities to explore, if not to appreciate, the significance that illnesses entail. Arthur Frank makes this point succinctly: "How medicine treats the body is an essential part of the story of illness, but it is never more than half of the story. The other half is the body itself. . . . These two stories, the story of *medicine taking the body as its territory*, and the story of *learning to wonder at the body itself*, can only be told together, because illness is both stories at once."[52] That's one reason why, when medicine downgrades healing from a central concept to an ancillary effect, it has such a deleterious impact on us: its absence from the stories we use to make sense of our experiences prompts us to pass over powerful possibilities toward which we, as living organisms, nonetheless tend (until we don't, and then we die).

By another twist of fate—that ultimately proved as surprising and life transforming to me as spontaneously slipping into trances—during my hospitalization at Stanford I began to think about how I thought about my illness for the first time and to consider how much my thinking had been shaped by the ways medicine thinks about disease. The prompt for this new reflection came from the example of the French thinker Michel Foucault. Because I wasn't able to go to classes during those months in the hospital, my advisor allowed me to do a directed reading on Foucault's works instead. One of the most famous intellectuals of the twentieth century, Foucault held a chair at the Collège de France that allowed him incredible latitude to explore what he called "the history of systems of thought." Needless to say, Foucault's project was complex and resists easy summary; nevertheless, another of the twentieth century's great thinkers, his erstwhile friend Gilles Deleuze, summed it up succinctly: "Only one thing has ever interested Foucault: What does it mean to think."[53] After decades of reading and rereading his writings, I might put it slightly differently: "Only one thing has ever interested Foucault: How does thinking matter?"

Either way, it's important to underscore that for Foucault, *thinking* does not refer to cerebral activity per se. It does not refer to the electrochemical processes that take place in our gray matter, nor does it name our capacity for cogitation or cognition in general. Instead, for Foucault, thinking gestures toward the possibility of reconsidering not only what one has thought before but also what one has taken for granted (perhaps by not thinking about it) in order to consider it otherwise. Foucault affirms that either thinking transforms us or else it is not really thinking at all: "Thought is not what inhabits a certain conduct and gives it its meaning; rather, it is what allows one to step back from this way of acting or reacting, to present it to oneself as an object of thought and to question it as to its meaning, its conditions, and its goals. Thought is freedom in relation to what one does, the motion by which one detaches from it, establishes it as an object, and reflects on it as a problem."[54]

Thought, in Foucault's perspective, introduces a distance, a detachment, a hesitation, a stutter, a pause, or even a swerve, into our habitual ways of making meaning from—or ascribing meaning to—our conduct. Such modulations in our usual manner of meaning making can manifest new potentials. They can reveal not only that our habitual behaviors might not be necessary, but that in fact they might restrict or conflict with our abilities to affirm our highest values or realize our fondest desires. Rather than repeating what we think we already know, thinking thus takes our familiar forms of thought as problems. It questions that which seemed to go without question in order to open up alternatives that do not and cannot appear until such questions get asked. That is why Foucault regards thinking as "freedom in relation to what one does."

Foucault thought of thinking as an event—that is, as something that takes place in time and that can change the times in which it takes place. Moreover, by thinking of thinking as an event, he understood his own work as troubling the self-evidence of what we take to be most self-evident about our lives, a process he referred to as "eventualization": "I am trying to work in the direction of what one might call 'eventualization.' . . . What do I mean by this term? First of all, a breach of self-evidence. . . . To show that things 'weren't as necessary as all that.'"[55] In pursuing this defamiliarizing intellectual practice, Foucault positioned himself primarily as a teacher who tried to open people to new ways of thinking and living. In an interview he gave two years before he died of AIDS in 1984, he affirmed that his aim was "to show people that they are much freer than they feel, that people accept as truth, as evidence, some themes which have been built up at a certain moment during history, and that this so-called evidence can be criticized and destroyed. To change something in the minds of people—that is the role of an intellectual."[56]

Of course, changing minds can also involve changing lives. It's what many of us who are teachers aspire to do. At its best, teaching does not just inculcate new skills and knowledge, although there's definitely some of that going on. Good teaching also helps students learn to ask productive questions, ones that might enable them to pursue new forms of thinking, and in the process create new forms of living.[57] Since I am a teacher, and have been one for almost four decades, Foucault's insights have given me much inspiration over the years. All teachers have had teachers of some sort or another. Foucault was one of my main teachers, although I knew him only through his writings. Nevertheless, discovering his thinking while lying in my hospital bed changed my life, and forty years later it still inspires me as I teach and as I write.[58] It's why I hope that by "eventualizing" what medicine knows—and what it doesn't know—this book might open up new possibilities for some of its readers for how they experience illness and healing, "to show that things 'weren't as necessary as all that.'"

$$\oint$$

In one of his earliest books, *The Birth of the Clinic: An Archaeology of Medical Perception,* Foucault meditates on how medicine became modern by "open[ing] up a few corpses" (mentioned above). Reading this text while confined to the clinic radically rearranged my thinking about what was happening to me in the Hoover Pavilion. Moreover, it gave me a new frame of reference from which to consider not only the things doctors had been telling me about my illness for the previous decade but also the things they did not and could not tell me.

*The Birth of the Clinic* traces the historical development of clinical medicine, which is the kind of medicine carried out in teaching hospitals like Stanford. Foucault suggests that during the late eighteenth and early nineteenth centuries, new ways of seeing and knowing emerged from the clinic that simultaneously introduced new ways to make sense of disease and to practice medicine. In the clinic, physicians began to introduce new protocols that led them to perceive their patients' afflictions as pathological manifestations of bodily matter. As a result, they began to see their patients not only as suffering people but also as sets of personified symptoms (a perspective familiar to us from hospital shows on TV: e.g., "Code Blue, the cardiac arrest in room 3 is crashing"). As Foucault put it, "Paradoxically in relation to what he is suffering from, the patient is only an external fact; the medical reading must take him into account only to place him in parentheses."[59] This purview in turn provided evidence of the deeper bodily transformations that diseases now appeared to manifest:

> In the anatamo-clinical experience, the medical eye must see the illness spread before it horizontally, and vertically graded in depth, as it penetrates into the body, advances into its bulk, as it circumvents or lifts its masses, as it descends into its depths. . . . [Disease] is no longer a pathological species inserting itself into the body wherever possible; it is the body itself that has become ill. . . . Disease loses its old status as an accident, and takes on the internal constant, mobile dimension of the relation between life and death. It is not because he falls ill that man dies; fundamentally, it is because he may die that he falls ill.[60]

According to Foucault, medicine's investment in disease's inexorability underwrites its modern manifestations. Instead of constituting a cruel twist of fate, or an unfortunate unbalancing of elements, or an act of God, modern medical pathology presents itself to us as the body gone awry. Hence, in the clinic, diseases began to appear as substantial transformations of the flesh, or lesions, that reveal the constant work of death within us.[61]

That is certainly how I had come to understand my own relation to Crohn's, especially after my near-death encounter. Yet my experience of radical illness followed by radical healing also confused these convictions. That's why Foucault's analysis spurred me to scrutinize the unspoken suppositions that suffused my relations with the doctors, residents, and interns who trooped through my room every day. It also aided me in assessing the assumptions that were altering my tissues on cellular, molecular, and subatomic levels via all the drugs that were being pumped into me. "My" disease, I slowly began to realize, was not really mine at all. It actually belonged to the gastroenterologists, pathologists, hematologists, radiologists, surgeons, imaging technologists, and so forth who viewed the vital-substance-that-I-took-to-be-me as both the source and the site of my affliction. From them, I had learned that there was something wrong *with* me because there was something wrong *in* me, and vice versa. Moreover, this wrongness was not just accidental, not just an inessential or unfortunate circumstance, but rather it revealed an irreducible flaw in my being: the fact that I was born to die. Crohn's disease, like all disease according to the anatamo-clinical framework, foretold my death even as my doctors sought to save my life (for the moment).

Redefining disease as in-depth pathology helped clinical medicine refine its diagnostic disposition, foreshadowing the diverse developments that characterize our contemporary medical-industrial complex. Until the end of the eighteenth century, hospitals had been religious refuges that indiscriminately amassed the indigent, aged, ill, insane, homeless, and hopeless. However, in that century's last decades, the hospital began to distinguish among these species of sufferers. It thereby began to reimagine itself not as a refuge of last resort (like the "last almshouse in America" where Victoria Sweet practiced) but as a "curing machine," *un machine à guérir* in Foucault's telling phrase.[62] This shift in mission turned out to have significant therapeutic consequences in the long term; however, in the short term it worked much more to medicine's benefit than to that of its patients. For, whatever curative enhancements this change in medical thought and practice enabled (which were not many at the time), the new clinical hospital more effectively served medicine as a pseudolaboratory.

As hospitals began to gather a range of suffering patients in one place, they allowed medicine to use them to accumulate data that it could then construe as evidence for medical hypotheses, as well as to provide cases from which doctors in training could learn. (This principle still holds in teaching hospitals like Stanford.) Conversely, since most clinical patients were poor, their subsidized care (such as it was) obliged them to serve as experimental subjects and/or teaching examples. Moreover, if and when they died, their corpses would pay off their debts in full. Subject to autopsy, these former bearers of symptoms transformed under the dissecting scalpel into the natural materials for scientific exploration. As physicians cut through these bodies, seeking evidence about the nature of the diseases that had killed them, the dead flesh seemed to reveal something true about the living organisms that they once were. This new medical enterprise, called pathological anatomy, institutionalized the requirement to "open up a few corpses" in order to generate positive knowledge about disease, so that henceforth "it is at death that disease and life speak their truth."[63]

Medicine first evinced its scientific ethos, then, not by laboratory experimentation, but by trying to correlate the symptoms it discerned in a population of living patients—which hospital clinics presented in abundance—with the lesions disclosed when their dead bodies were dissected. In so doing, clinical medicine forged the idea that these lesions represent the site—or "seat" (*siège*) as it appears in French—of the disease and concomitantly introduced the premise that disease as such exists apart from any particular bodily locations where it might happen to take place. We call this dual approach an "ontological theory of disease." (Consider one recent example: although "COVID-19" encompasses a wide range of possible symptoms—from none to mild to severe to fatal—which affect different tissues and organ systems, including the lungs, intestines, kidneys, and brains, as well as toes, sometimes provoking deadly immunological reactions called "cytokine storms," the now sadly familiar term supposes that a singular infectious disease, correlated with a coronavirus, SARS-CoV-2, somehow exists above and beyond everybody—or indeed every body—who currently has, or has had, it.[64]) By defining disease as an ontological object subject to analytic investigation, this clinical reframing opened disease to a scientific analysis that had eluded medicine until that point. Moreover, the correspondences that clinical medicine created between the symptoms evinced in a patient population and the lesions found in their corpses made it possible to statistically analyze patterns of disease correlations across large numbers of people. It thereby implied that underlying the experience of disease there exists a calculable—if not predictable—pattern, and thus it affirmed that disease, like any other natural phenomenon, must submit to mathematical accountability. Taken together, the ontological theory of disease and the statistical representations of their effects induced medicine to regard itself as scientifically inclined. With this turn toward a more scientific way of knowing, medicine no doubt tried to make its knowledge claims more effective; yet it did so not merely to make them more reliable—which clinical medicine did not really do for quite some time—but also to make them more respectable, and possibly more profitable.

But what does the clinic tell us about healing? Alas, not so much. Insofar as it professionally invests in death as the raison d'être of disease, as disease's main motivation, medicine's clinical modality made healing harder to fathom. By focusing its attention on pathology, the clinic made disease substantial in a way it had never been before. Clinically speaking, or at least speaking in a clinical context, our diseases are us, while most other dimensions of our lives recede toward the vanishing point of our diagnosis. Yet, while reading Foucault in the hospital, I suddenly started to suspect that there was more to my illness than this pathological perspective permitted. At the time, I didn't have much more than a faint glimmer of what this new way of thinking might involve. Although the trances indicated other ways of experiencing Crohn's might be possible, if not necessary, I didn't yet know how to ask questions about them in a productive way. Yet just as the healing intelligence evinced by my cells and molecules intimated that I was more than I knew, Foucault's text invited me to reconsider what I thought I already knew about Crohn's, since this knowledge was entirely embedded in a clinical frame of reference. It took me a while to take up that invitation, and it turned out that in order to do so, I needed the support and encouragement of others who had also negotiated the clinical model and lived to tell the tale. The following chapters describe the steep learning curve I had to ascend in order to find enough freedom from Crohn's clinical classification to embrace healing—rather than disease—as my destiny.

I now believe that the events I came to know as "having Crohn's disease" not only entailed a lot of painful shit but also provided an opportunity to consider my life—if not life itself—completely otherwise. Instead of an acute affliction, from the perspective of healing, having Crohn's involved passing through a number of healing crises, which, although often dramatic and frightening, eventually challenged me to recognize that a tendency toward healing, as well as toward death, moved within me. These critical events pulled me up short and interrupted my self-narrative, completely disrupting what I had previously called my "self." They challenged me to revise my story, not only about who I am but also about *what* I am—not to mention about what an *I* might be in the first place. By thinking though my illness differently, by reflecting on the experiences it provoked, and by ruminating not only on the ways that medicine had encouraged me to know it but also on the limits folded within this knowledge, I began to incorporate it differently. And when I actually took that to heart, it gave me more courage to deal with the shit that life throws out. *On Learning to Heal* draws on these experiences to affirm the possibility that with enough support and encouragement—which, of course, includes having the necessary economic, political, psychological, social, and spiritual resources—we might be able to heal because we tend to heal, even though in the end we will all also die. It shares some hard-won lessons that changed my thinking about living *and* healing with a chronic illness and that thereby changed how I live that illness and how it lives in me as well.

# TWO

## We Are More Complicated Than We Know

We are unknown to ourselves, we men of knowledge, and with good reason.
—FRIEDRICH NIETZSCHE, *On the Genealogy of Morality* (1887)

Living with a chronic illness involves a lot of not-knowing and even more complications. For example: Who knows when or how a chronic illness begins? Is there a moment when an illness becomes chronic? Or does chronicity instead conceal a temporal convolution that entirely changes one's "life-time"— that is, one's awareness of one's life as both temporal and temporary? After all, in ancient Greek myth, Kronos (whose name *chronic* immortalizes) was the leader of the Titans and the ruler of time, especially time viewed in its violent and devouring valence.[1] In my case, time chronically cracked open during a cross-country trip in the family station wagon. In retrospect, I realize that intimations of incontinence must have existed before I or my parents recognized something was seriously amiss. However, because we all packed into the car without giving it a second thought, nothing must have seemed too out of whack. While I do remember that by the end of eighth grade I was already putting in a fair amount of toilet time, before we backed out of the driveway this was just attributed to my well-established tendencies toward anxiety. (Compounded no doubt by the dim but dilating awareness of my attraction to other boys as puberty pursued me, but that's another realization that only occurred retrospectively.) It wasn't until we hit middle America that the insistence of my intestinal insurrection became inescapable. Nothing like having flagrant diarrhea during July and August, while trapped in a dark blue station wagon with vinyl seats and no air conditioning traveling on interstates where rest stops are few and far between, to make you appreciate just how excruciating time's expanses can be.

Needless to say, toilet training is sorely tested in such circumstances, and sometimes you fail the test. Repeatedly. Unfortunately, even the best training doesn't always prepare you for all the shit that can happen. For most of the eight-week ordeal, my parents tried to stanch the flow of my shit by conventional means: buying over-the-counter antidiarrhea medicines; making me eat rice, bananas, and clear chicken broth; forcing me to drink copious quantities of liquid; and so on. Twice they took me to emergency rooms where more powerful potions were prescribed, although with no significant success. My stealthy shit seemed undaunted by the chalky elixirs that the ER doctors threw at it, and it could slip by even the most staunchly guarded sphincters without the slightest difficulty. Consequently, I spent most of my time on the road either dozing in the front seat, exhausted by dehydration and increasing malnutrition, or frantically trying to maintain bowel control until I could get my father to pull over at the nearest available toilet, outhouse, or clump of bushes where I could relieve myself. By the time that happened, it usually felt like I was expelling my guts.

I'm sure my parents were worried about me. However, they were busy circumnavigating North America with four adolescent boys (my two younger brothers, my older cousin, and me) ages fourteen, thirteen, twelve, and eleven, on what was supposed to be an enlightening educational experience. Given my parents' proclivities, this involved visits to urban ghettos and Native American reservations (Mom) as well as trips to national parks, especially those with geological or paleontological significance (Dad). In between these destinations, because the diversions offered by digital devices did not yet exist, we only had AM/FM radio to mediate all the enforced family time (yet another chronic condition?). In light of the extreme challenges that so much unmediated togetherness presented, my parents' prime objective was obviously to get us there and back in one piece before we killed each other. Despite the fact that we all survived the familiar fighting, the transcontinental trip nevertheless took a toll on me. By the time we arrived back at my grandmother's apartment to drop my cousin off, I must have been a mere shadow of my former self, because the moment my grandmother opened the door, she started screaming.

After that, I began going to a lot of doctors. Luckily my father's job came with a very good health insurance plan, so paying for these visits was not an obstacle (as it could have been for many, given that the United States does not have universal health care). The first was my pediatrician, who agreed that this wasn't your everyday diarrhea and sent me to an internist at the local hospital where I was born. After some initial testing, blood work, and X-rays (the first of my many upper GI series and barium enemas), the internist prescribed a weird foam that I had to inject into my anus twice a day. When that proved unhelpful, he in turn sent me to a "famous gastroenterologist" at Johns Hopkins, about thirty miles from where I lived. The famous gastroenterologist read the files forwarded from the internist, looked at the X-rays that we'd carefully transported in their oversized manila envelope, and did a cursory physical exam by brusquely palpating my abdomen while inquiring, "Does this hurt?"; "Does this hurt?"; "Does this?" (Answer: "Yes, asshole.") He then told my parents I needed to be hospitalized immediately and referred me to yet another gastroenterologist, his former resident, who worked at the nearby University of Maryland hospital. At this point, my mother had to break it to me that I was really sick, that the doctors didn't know what was wrong with me, and that rather than starting high school with the rest of my cohort, I'd be going to the hospital.

Living with a chronic illness is complicated; trying to get a diagnosis is just the beginning. Before a diagnosis, you might have excruciating experiences that explode life as you knew it, but you don't know what's happening (not that we ever really *know* what's happening). Sometimes your doctors don't immediately know either. In those days, you could still be admitted to the hospital for diagnostic testing, a practice that current reimbursement procedures have pretty much curtailed. In my case, it took another month or so of testing and imaging for things to come into focus, during which time no orifice was left unprobed. Between the barium swallows and enemas, the endoscopes and fluoroscopes, the sigmoidoscopes and colonoscopes, I didn't know which end was up. Needless to say, the diagnostic search that sets medicine in motion requires a body to disclose its deepest secrets—often thanks to various imaging technologies.[2] Alas, because we're fairly opaque beings, these investigations can occasion varying degrees of "discomfort"—medical code for pain (don't say no one ever warned you). And when you're hospitalized for periods of time, such discomfort becomes a constant companion.

After a few weeks of intense interrogation, the unknown dissidents destroying my digestion capitulated to my doctors' demands to divulge their identity. In this way, I was really lucky. Some people spend years in search of an adequate diagnosis; some never get one at all. But after evaluating the multitude of X-rays, blood work, biopsies, and scans that cast light upon my intestinal turmoil, my new gastroenterologist confidently conferred a name upon my shitty predicament: Crohn's. When the team of doctors and doctors-in-training crowded into my narrow hospital room to make their official pronouncement—and, since this was a teaching hospital, there was always a team—the name meant nothing to me. All I could infer from the diagnosis was that they now knew something about what was happening to me (something that I didn't) and that perhaps as a result there was something they could do to stop it. The naming ceremony—or "the reveal," as they might say on reality TV—seemed to justify my hope that if my inner turbulence conformed to my doctors' ways of knowing, it would be tamed by their treatments. At the time, I didn't know enough about either Crohn's disease in particular or illness in general to know that wasn't going to happen.

These days, an adolescent presenting with fulminating diarrhea, acute intestinal cramps, and rapid wasting might not have to wait long for a diagnosis. However, in the early 1970s Crohn's was still primarily associated with adult Jews rather than pubescent ones. Indeed, for a little while I thought they said I had "Crone's disease"; now I think it may have precociously turned me into a crone. Be that as it may, before the diagnosis, "my problem" appeared first and foremost in the form of fecal flash floods. Why shit oozed from my rectum; why everything I put in my mouth transited my intestines and then promptly propelled out my ass; why I suffered intestinal spasms that left me doubled over in pain and gasping for breath—none of these made any particular sense. After the doctors dubbed the deluge of diarrhea "Crohn's disease," it adopted a different demeanor. Now all the shit happening to me represented a "disease" that I "had." That meant—I mistakenly thought at the time—it had a cause and that cause could be treated, and I would be cured. (Cue triumphal music.) Perhaps because I was only thirteen and spent a lot of my time living in books, I initially received "Crohn's" as if it were a medical-magical talisman bestowed by my doctors to ward off my body's untoward, and frequently unexpected, irruptions. I accepted that the name contained my problem—or at least I hoped it would, because the shit itself seemed uncontainable.

If the diagnosis appeared to give my incontinence some shape, some definition, some boundaries, it also gave me some expectations, some ideas, some stories to live by. Of course, what I thought "Crohn's" meant and what my doctors meant by it did not exactly coincide. My Crohn's was not their Crohn's and vice versa. To me, Crohn's disease named the source from which all my shit flowed. The specificity of the words themselves made it seem as if it was the province of a particular physician (Dr. Crohn), and somehow this proprietary provenance appeared to promise an end to my body's ungovernability. (As we'll see shortly, the promise of governability lies at the root of all medicine and, hence, at the heart of the doctor-patient pas de deux.) If Crohn's was literally a pain in my ass, the fact that it could be named as such suggested to me that the shitty situation might be medically conjured away. After all, wasn't that what both medical knowledge and magical words were supposed to do?

In contrast to my wishful thinking, to my doctors Crohn's disease denominated a complicated, not entirely well understood form of autoimmune dysregulation that had impaired my small intestine's normal function, inflaming its lining and disrupting its ability to absorb nutrients from food. Moreover, they proposed that this pathological propensity could be managed by powerful, toxic pharmaceuticals that would help mitigate the inflammation.[3] Theoretically, these medications would dampen my distressing symptoms by modulating my adverse immune response to my own tissues. Regrettably, this worked better in theory than in practice. Clearly, what I naively thought my doctors meant and what they thought they meant inhabited entirely different worlds. Of course, this isn't very surprising, since a diagnosis performs different kinds of work for a doctor and for a patient. It matters differently to each.

Diagnosis involves living under a medical description. If you're lucky, and such a thing exists, it can mean living under a medical prescription as well. Diagnosis inscribes an illness upon you by anointing you with its name. ("I baptize thee with the name of Crohn's.") It signs its name upon you and thereby assigns its name to you. It writes itself both in your medical records and on your body. I mean this quite literally, since in Latin the *script* that lingers at the roots of *description*, *prescription*, and *inscription* means "to write." Mobilizing its many scripts, medical knowledge converts the volatile and vulnerable organisms that we are into vital surfaces upon which it etches its therapeutic thoughts. These thoughts then appear as words, such as "Crohn's disease," "terminal ileitis," "regional enteritis," "abnormal inflammation," "autoimmunity," "immunosuppression," words that construct correlations between test results and symptoms. Since test results usually contain numbers or images whose significance can only be ascertained by assigning values to them, such evaluations always entail interpretation.[4] Once delivered in the form of a diagnosis, these vital interpretations then enter into our experiences of illness as ways of both grasping and communicating their consequences.

Interpretation is necessary because organisms don't naturally speak our language, or any language for that matter. Although bioscience has spent much of the last seventy-five years depicting DNA in terms of coding and transcription (yet another bioscientific script), implying that language-like activities underwrite the existence of all living beings, these ideas are in fact metaphors, attributed to vital phenomena precisely because the phenomena themselves do not and cannot speak to us directly.[5] Indeed, as Michel Foucault reflected, "It is not natural for nature to be known."[6] Medicine modifies the muteness of our molecules, cells, tissues, and organs by manufacturing links that span the incommensurability between their modes of mattering and our ways of deciding what matters to us. These links are what we call metaphors. Metaphors create connections between things that are naturally distinct, bringing them into proximity, inducing fields of tension between them from which new meanings can emerge.[7]

In order to achieve such metaphorical conversions, biomedical thinking must translate the transformations of matter and energy that animate our cells and molecules into its own languages. If these no longer include the Latin and Greek that all prospective doctors once had to learn, then they certainly involve the biochemistry and genomics that all physicians and bioscientists must now master. Unfortunately for us, neither illnesses nor organisms reveal their significance immediately. This is, after all, why we ask medicine to speak for them. Biomedicine attempts to parse the natural idioms of our vulnerable organisms in order to render their (dys)functions familiar—or least hopefully familiar to our physicians (while we keep our fingers crossed). It believes that by making our symptoms legible and by deciphering their significance, its interpretive interventions may, in turn, underwrite effective therapies. This is what medicine does because this is what medicine is. It's what has made medicine "medicine" ever since medicine first began to be medicine more than twenty-five hundred years ago.

Medicine was certainly not the first and is still not the only form of healing therapy. Indeed, in order to become "medicine," it had to distinguish itself from the other therapeutic practices that already existed, which it began to do sometime around the fifth century BCE. Over the next two and a half millennia, medicine secured a significant share of the therapy market, edging out its chief competitors: magicians, root cutters, temple priests, doctor-prophets, purifiers, drug vendors, herbalists, and the like (not to mention the gods). Since licensing authorities did not yet exist to discriminate among these practitioners—as they wouldn't for the next two millennia—medicine's early prospects depended entirely on its ability to persuade people of its preeminence. In other words, as a therapeutic intervention, medicine had to prove that its performance would be profitable to all concerned.[8] *Therapy* comes from a Greek verb that has a range of meanings: to attend to, to be of service to, to heed, to devote oneself to, to cultivate, and eventually it comes to mean to treat medically.[9] Underlying all these senses is the notion of therapy as a way of looking after, tending to, and caring for. Therapy initially referred to a range of services or attentions bestowed upon someone or something, including gods, parents, children, plants, animals, and temples; however, following the birth of medicine, therapy expanded its purview to include medical and surgical treatments or cures as well. In the ensuing centuries, medicine's knowing devotions declared it a distinctive form of therapy, predicated on a singular form of *savoir faire*, one in which doing (*faire*) was tied to knowing (*savoir*) in very tangible ways. By knitting knowing and doing together, medicine rooted its therapeutic rationale in the sphere of knowledge. Ever since, medicine's knowing ways have defined its stock-in-trade. Remember: *diagnosis* means "by way of knowledge."

Medicine has always insisted that its competitive advantages follow from its devotion to knowing. Forswearing allegiance to gods, spirits, disembodied powers, or other immaterial forces, medicine takes knowing per se as its forte. Whether or not it can actually do anything to relieve our suffering, medicine has always assumed that knowing and naming—which diagnosis demands—have value, even if they don't actually have curative consequences. Thus, it assumes that when it comes to disease, if not healing, knowing makes a deliberate difference. This assumption founds itself on the fact that a diagnosis not only designates a disorder, but in so doing it differentiates that disorder from other disorders. This differentiation determines the diagnosis. In other words, medical diagnosis is a differential diagnosis. In order to know a disease, and thereby name it, you first have to define it. This means you have to delimit it, separating it from whatever it is not.

Since its advent in ancient Greece, making such a diagnostic distinction has constituted the decisive act of medical judgment. Indeed, medicine developed the possibility for therapeutic knowing by cultivating these practices of exclusion and decision, which it then touted as the basis for its technical acumen. As a consequence, the ability to diagnostically differentiate diseases came to distinguish one doctor's skills from another's. This diagnostic difference in turn established reputations (aka income-generating potentials). The great Hippocrates himself supposedly became history's founding physician only after triumphing in a public contest to determine who could diagnose most deftly. In the long run, his triumph turns out to have triggered an important transition in Western therapeutics.

Diagnosticians, whom we also call physicians, set out to enlighten us about what we don't know about ourselves, or at least about the shit that is happening to us. This enlightened and enlightening knowledge not only orients the physician's actions on our behalf; it also conjures different foreseeable futures for us. Medicine labels these future fictions *prognoses* (a Latin translation of a Greek word meaning "to know beforehand").[10] Prognoses fabricate feasible, though never unfailing, scenarios by deducing probable developments from diagnoses. We might think of a prognosis as a diagnosis played in fast forward, scanning through multiple selected scenarios at the same time in order to pick out the most plausible narrative possibilities. As such, prognoses support medicine's claims that knowing can allow it to glimpse our futures, if not change them. From its inception, this prognostic proclivity has served as medicine's main means of marketing, as the Hippocratic text titled *Prognostic* underscored more than twenty-two hundred years ago:

> It seems to me best for a physician to try to understand things in advance. For if he knows them in advance and predicts in the presence of his patients what is happening, what has happened, and what will happen (to the extent that these things were left out of the patient's original account), the more he will be believed to know his patients' real situations, so that people will dare to place themselves in the doctor's hands. What's more, he will give the best treatment if he knows in advance what will happen on the basis of present symptoms.[11]

By offering diagnoses and prognoses, medicine tries to anticipate a patient's prospects before they come to pass. If possible, its treatments then attempt to alter these (anticipated) temporal trajectories. Time is thus of the essence for medicine. Its ability to prognosticate depends upon its ability to extrapolate from present circumstances in order to predict what is not yet manifest but still likely to come. Hence, by applying its knowledge to the things that are happening now, medicine seeks not only to ameliorate our immediate suffering but also to preempt even more of it later. In ancient Greek medicine, a physician's diagnostic abilities proved themselves by discerning the most auspicious times to intervene. These moments were called crises. In Greek, *krisis* means judgment, decision, or separation; choice, election, or interpretation; event, issue to be decided; and subsequently came to mean turning point or sudden change in a disease.[12] Crisis thus denoted the decisive instance in which a physician must choose either to act or to refrain from acting in order to redirect the development of a disease.

Deciding upon the proper time to act, as well as determining what to do in the event, proved critical for medicine's entangled therapeutic, epistemological, and commercial aspirations. By orienting its knowledge in and through time in order to anticipate (if not alter) patients' prospects, medicine made cri-sis management its métier. Crises cry out for medical attention. Consequently, crises constitute medicine's motivating moments—although ones that do not, in themselves, belong to its domain. Time, after all, belongs to no one. (This might be one reason why medicine is still better at treating critical rather than chronic conditions.) When physicians deploy their knowledge to depict the dangers that loom before us, they seek to convert such crises into chances to change our fates. By detecting where—or rather when—the descent toward death diverges from the road back to life, medicine aspires to intervene criti-cally in order to decide *for* life and *against* death.

Yet, because medicine is by definition not magic, it works only by regulating our routines. In Hippocratic medicine, this regulation was called *dietetics* in Greek (from *diatata*, meaning way of living or mode of life) or *regimen* in Latin (from *rego*, to rule, to guide, lead, conduct, manage, direct, correct).[13] Along with pharmacopoeia and surgery, it constituted one of Greek medicine's three therapeutic domains. Underscoring medicine's initial (and enduring) invest-ments in this regulative propensity, the great twentieth-century linguist Émile Benveniste argued that the *med-* in *medicine* comes from an Indo-European root that simultaneously meant to judge, to govern, and to cure.[14] Sprouting from this seed syllable, medicine has always fused its modes of reflection with forms of authority. In other words, medicine as medicine puts its knowledge into therapeutic practice by deploying it authoritatively. Ever since we began to appeal to physicians to govern our behaviors, and to submit ourselves to their supervision, we have actively placed our faith in the power of their knowledge to rule us by judging, governing, and curing us.

For more than two and a half millennia, medicine has offered us its knowl-edge in exchange for our accepting this governing guidance. Knowing and governing have always constituted the two sides of medicine's power. In an-cient Greece, where it commenced, medicine invented this tangled technique, inaugurating it as something heretofore entirely unknown by constituting it as something that must be known, as Benveniste observed: "It appears that Indo-European 'medicine' supposes reflection, competence, and authority. The 'treatment' of illnesses mobilizes the same capacities, and demands the same kind of 'measures,' as the command of men or the practice of the judiciary. It is an entirely different thing than primitive medicine. . . . The doctor [*médecin*] no longer has anything to do with the magician; he is a man of thought."[15] Opposing itself to magic, or any other unknown and unknowable forces, med-ical thinking affirms itself as a reflective knowledge that claims the capacity to command others (much as the law and the military do). Hence, medicine offers itself as what, following Foucault, we might designate as a type of "governance," insofar as "to govern . . . is to structure the possible field of actions of others."[16] Medical governance calls us to conduct ourselves according to its rules through what it now calls compliance. It asks us to take our doctors' knowing to heart and to learn to live by it.

In offering the physician's vital knowledge as a governing regime, medicine frames how we come to know our own experiences of illness. It therefore informs not only how disease lives in us but also how we live through it—if we do. Governing through knowledge, medicine forswears any dependence on the mysterious powers, influences, and figures invoked by premedical protocols. (I mean *premedical* in the sense that we speak of thinkers before Socrates as pre-Socratic.) Instead, medicine commends itself to us by committing itself to careful knowing as its rationale. Thus, in ancient Greece, as *therapia* (treatment or care) began to become "medical," it sought to conduct the conduct of others through a "pre-*med*-itated" knowledge of disease that it claimed as its own.[17]

While waiting for a diagnosis, I spent a fair amount of time lying around the hospital. There are only so many tests that can be performed in a day, which left me with some free time. My private room was at the end of a long corridor in the old wing of the University of Maryland hospital, next to a solarium, where patients' families gathered to exchange bad news in hushed tones (which I could still overhear thanks to an acoustical quirk, probably having to do with the extremely high ceilings). Across the hall an old woman lay dying quietly. The nurses aimed their questions at her in strenuous voices, trying to pierce her profound deafness, if not her isolation—Did she want a pillow? Would she eat some of her meal? Did she need the bedpan? I never heard her reply. A week or two later, a doctor with some advanced and painful cancer moved into that room. When his angry yelling replaced her somber silence, I learned something significant about how different people approach death.

The only person around my age was the sixteen-year-old girl next door who had leukemia. Sometimes we'd watch TV together after visiting hours, when our mothers had both left for the night. A few months later, as I was convalescing at home, her mother called to say that she had passed away. The only other person I met on my wing was a twenty-something young woman who meticulously applied her makeup every day as she lounged on her mechanical bed. The magic of mascara and eyeliner—whose provocative powers she enthusiastically endorsed—made her seem terribly sophisticated to my thirteen-year-old eyes. She also had ulcerative colitis. Because we'd both been diagnosed with inflammatory bowel diseases, our mothers thought we'd enjoy chatting. One morning as I went past her room, it was empty. A few days later, as I went by, I heard inconsolable crying. In the interim, they'd taken out her colon. I'm sure losing a colon is never easy to bear. Yet something about the sounds of her sorrow signaled—even to my adolescent ears—that it wasn't just her colon that she grieved. I didn't have a clue as to what it might be, but I fervently hoped I wouldn't have to find out anytime soon.

Before my hospitalization I'd tried not to think much about death, let alone my own death. I was a pretty anxious child, and intimations of mortality could easily push me over the edge into full-fledged panic. To this day I don't watch violent movies. At that age, the theme song from Zsa Zsa Gabor's movie *Picture Mommy Dead*, a coyly lilting tune with morbid lyrics—"The worms crawl in / The worms crawl out / In your stomach / And out your mouth"—sparked nightmares. (Only years later did the movie's conspicuous campiness become clear to me.) Yet spending time around people actively dying left me curiously numb. I didn't—or couldn't—yet recognize myself in their place, so I closed my mind to them. I remember telling myself: I'm only thirteen. I'm too young to think about death—I'll deal with it when I'm in my twenties (which retrospectively turns out to have been a fateful thought). My plan mostly worked, except for one night, near the end of my hospital sojourn, when *In Cold Blood* appeared on the Late Night Movie. Emanating from the hulking black-and-white TV looming over my bed, death deviously defied my defenses. Maybe it was because I was high on my newly prescribed corticosteroids, but something about the unsuspecting family miserably murdered in their farmhouse, their sheer familiar terror, struck home. (By one of life's weird coincidences, years later the actress who played the terrified teenage daughter, murdered in the movie's first act, would marry one of my best friends.)

Mostly my death-defying took the form of reading thick nineteenth-century novels. The great thing about these tomes was not just their length, which promised prolonged respites from hospital routine, but their reliable resolutions. Whatever problems plagued the characters, you could usually trust that by the end they'd be settled and that for the most part these settlements would be satisfying (except for some of the French and Russian novels, which could be downers). Probably the pleasures of anticipated closure, even hundreds of pages in the future, unconsciously assuaged my uncertainties about my own story. While the medical team would come by every day to update us about my situation, for the first few weeks their inconclusive visits didn't mollify my anxiety much. Mostly they reported on the tests they'd just done and announced the new tests they wanted to perform. The next day an orderly would wheel me hither and thither through the corridors to some new equipment site where another assault on my as-yet intractable illness would be staged. The doctors' implacable quest for knowledge claimed my teenage body as its own. Sometimes when they described the indignities they planned to commit next, I'd say to myself: over my dead body. Nevertheless, somewhere below the surface of my consciousness, I also realized that this might be the very outcome they were trying to preempt.

$$\dagger$$

When I was first diagnosed with Crohn's disease, my doctors tried to explain it to me: Crohn's is an autoimmune illness, they said. Now for a thirteen-year-old I had a pretty big vocabulary, but *autoimmunity* wasn't one of my words, so they tried to break it down for me. First, they offered, "Well, it's like you're allergic to yourself." That seemed a bit fuzzy, so they added, "It's as if your body is rejecting part of itself." Despite the clarification I was still at sea, so they threw out one more image: "You're eating yourself alive." Okay, that stuck. Unfortunately, I lived with that image for a long time. The diagnosis didn't just tell me what Crohn's was, or what it did; it infected my relation to myself. Now, in addition to making me shit my pants and run screaming for the toilet at an instant's notice—exciting a deep envy of dogs, who could just squat on the street—Crohn's apparently troubled my ability to tolerate myself, or at least my "self." (As we'll discover in a bit, most immunologists hold that "self-tolerance" constitutes the basic immunological parameter whose breakdown precipitates autoimmune diseases.) Moreover, by introducing the idea that I was "allergic" to myself, or "rejecting myself," or "eating myself alive," the explanation of the diagnosis seemed to imply that I was, however inadvertently, the cause as well as the effect of my own distress. Did I just need to get over myself? Or, over my "self"? It was rather confusing.

Since I knew so little about Crohn's, I assumed my doctors must know everything about it, which turns out not to have been the case—and forty years later it is even less the case. Obviously, these days Crohn's constitutes a well-established clinical entity, supporting a thriving subfield in gastroenterology as well as a pharmaceutically funded patient advocacy organization, the Crohn's and Colitis Foundation, whose television ads you may have seen. Because it can now be treated with very expensive, and hence highly profitable, biologic medications called tumor necrosis factor inhibitors, like Remicade (infliximab) and Humira (adalimumab), as well as newer monoclonal antibodies like

Cosentyx (secukinumab), which binds to a proinflammatory cytokine, inter-leukin-17A, it also features widely in print, television, and digital media adver-tising.[18] Moreover, as the incidence of Crohn's increases around the world, the global marketing campaigns for these drugs have likewise helped expand its international recognition factor.[19] While not necessarily in the top ten of high-profile pathologies, Crohn's has nevertheless carved out a nice niche for itself in the pantheon of twenty-first-century digestive disorders. However, Crohn's has not always had such a prominent place in either medical or public awareness. Indeed, before 1932 it didn't exist as such. That is not to say that nobody, or no body, had ever manifested the shitty symptoms we now recognize as Crohn's. For example, some claim that Charles Darwin and Prince Albert, Queen Vic-toria's consort, both had Crohn's.[20] However, before Burrill Crohn along with coauthors Leon Ginzburg and Gordon Oppenheimer published their semi-nal essay "Regional Ileitis: A Pathologic and Clinical Entity" in the *Journal of the American Medical Association*, the constellation of symptoms now called Crohn's did not cohere clinically.[21] Only after they were proclaimed symptoms of a new intestinal disorder did they take on their significance as signs of an underlying yet unknown pathology.

The first framing of Crohn's or, to use Burrill Crohn's favored terminology, regional ileitis mainly endeavored to differentiate this diagnosis from ulcerative colitis, which had been denominated as a disease during the late nineteenth century.[22] Thus, Dr. Crohn's initial intervention was largely classificatory or, in medicine's idiom, nosological. What sparked the pathology or why it developed was—and still is—far from clear, and treatment, as Crohn remarked, "is purely palliative and supportive." If the situation got too bad or too painful (e.g., when intestines got blocked or hemorrhaging occurred), Crohn suggested that "the proper approach to a complete cure is by surgical resection of the diseased seg-ment."[23] Twenty years after this seminal essay appeared, Crohn and his protégé, Henry Janowitz—the renowned gastroenterologist (and father of my friend Annie) who first asked me how Crohn's had affected my life—reported that the intervening decades had both produced more empirical evidence to verify the disease's differential determination (i.e., verifying that it remained significantly different from ulcerative colitis) and expanded the range of tissues it affected (from just the small bowel to the entire digestive tract). Yet, despite these seeming ad-vances, they also conceded, "there is no specific therapy for regional enteritis [yet another name for the disease] and all available measures are strictly supportive."[24]

Although diagnostic and therapeutic options have certainly multiplied in the seventy-five years since Crohn and Janowitz reflected on early clinical inter-ventions, specific therapies for Crohn's still do not exist, and available measures are still strictly supportive. Indeed, in the 1980s, when I first consulted Dr. J. in his Fifth Avenue office—which had been Dr. Crohn's office before him—he said something like that to me, if not using those exact words. Since then, I've read or heard versions of this statement so many times I've come to think of it as medicine's "Crohn's refrain." Hence, while we could say options for treating Crohn's have progressed, in the sense that they can more effectively dampen inflammation for longer periods of time while inducing somewhat fewer toxic side effects, a compelling elucidation of Crohn's remains elusive. In part, this elusiveness endures because the ongoing bioscientific elaboration of gastro-intestinal phenomena has revealed that the gut's cellular and biomolecular processes are far more complex than previously imagined. Given the current mappings of the labyrinthine landscape within which Crohn's takes place, any new explanations for the disease must include (at the very least) genetic, immu-nological, neurological, endocrinological, and bacteriological entanglements. To which we might want to add: environmental, sanitary, social, psychic, sexual, gendered, racialized, class-differentiated, and access-to-health-care-stratified variables—though medicine mostly doesn't go there (yet).

Consider just two of the discoveries with which attempts to understand Crohn's must now contend. First, the enteric nervous system: evidence for the enteric nervous system—sometimes called the "brain in the gut" or the "second brain"—has existed since the 1920s. Yet because of the dominance of brain-centric ideologies of neurological function, its significance only became more widely appreciated in the 1980s, around the time that selective serotonin reuptake in-hibitors (SSRIs) began to be used as antidepressants. The side effects of SSRIs regularly involved intestinal issues (diarrhea, constipation, bloating, nausea, etc.) that in turn raised the question, why? Investigating this digestive dilemma, stud-ies showed that the small intestine contains most of the same neuroreceptors as the brain and that it makes most of the same neurotransmitters (including up to 90 percent of the serotonin whose reuptake we now spend so much money trying to inhibit).[25] The interplay of chemical and electrical signals between the gut and the brain challenges brain-centered notions of neurophysiology and has led to greater acceptance of the idea that complex "cross-talk" between the two "brains" affects how we think and feel—perhaps providing empirical evidence for what people used to call "gut instinct" or even "gut wisdom."[26]

Second, our commensal microbes: thanks to the invention of new biotech-nologies, particularly high-throughput genetic sequencing that can rapidly analyze large quantities of genetic material, the commensal bacteria, viruses, and fungi that inhabit our guts are beginning to be identified and analyzed. As a consequence, we can now appreciate that the gut's evolving microbial ecology not only informs its functions—and dysfunctions—but also biochemically interacts with both the enteric nervous system and the enteric immune system, which reciprocally modulate the microbiome. In turn, the enteric immune system, which contains 70 to 80 percent of the entire population of our immune cells, continuously attempts to regulate this thriving threshold where inside/outside and self/other both coincide and collide. Collectively, these diverse biomolecular and cellular dynamics describe an exciting enteric environment replete with multidirectional signaling patterns whose diverse constituents defy easy comprehension.[27]

However, when Burrill Crohn first described the disease that would take his name, none of this was known, and doctors still understood the gastrointestinal tract as a quasi-autonomous organ system within the human body. We now understand that this segmented schema does not encompass the complications that unfold within either digestive function or dysfunction. Today, even keeping track of all the precipitating factors that Crohn's puts into play requires some very fancy footwork. Attempting to encompass this complex choreography, one recent medical review characterized Crohn's as "a polygenetic immune disorder with complex multifactorial etiology, generally arising in susceptible individuals in whom, upon environmental triggers, a sustained, disturbed, and deleterious mucosal immune reaction is provoked towards commensal bacteria."[28] As the serpentine syntax of this sentence suggests, contemporary medical thinking about Crohn's involves highly complicated interactions among genetic, immunological, intestinal, microbial, and environmental factors. However, when I was first diagnosed in the early 1970s, these complications had yet to reveal their full consequences, and most gastroenterologists—including mine—stressed the immunological implications over the others, presenting Crohn's primarily as an autoimmune disease.

In other words, they believed that for some (still) unknown reason, the immune system misrecognizes the lining of the gut as if it were foreign tissue—or as what immunology calls "not-self"—and defends against it. According to this explanation, autoantibodies generated by the acquired immune system react to the body's own tissues as if these tissues had somehow mysteriously appeared from elsewhere. Thus, rather than protect us from not-self, as the immune system has purportedly evolved to do, in autoimmune diseases our misguided immune defenses (purportedly) seek the wrong targets. When this happens, the immunological "friendly fire" can inflict heavy collateral damage or, indeed, initiate a "chronic immunological civil war."[29] According to this scenario, Crohn's occurs when the immune system mistakenly homes in on the cells lining the intestinal tract, stoking shitstorms in its wake.[30]

Immunological explanations for Crohn's still prevail, albeit while also attempting to acknowledge other agents like our genes, our intestinal microbiota, and our enteric nervous and immune system interactions.[31] Yet today there is less, rather than more, certainty about them. Not only do the multifactorial theories of digestive function expand the etiological focus beyond autoimmune explanations per se, but they alter immune thinking about Crohn's itself. Some recent theories suggest that instead of autoimmunity, Crohn's manifests a type of immunodeficiency (the antithesis of autoimmunity, which could be described as a kind of "immunoexcess").[32] Others propose that it represents a chronic autoinflammatory condition (a concept that refers to the damaging effects induced by innate rather than acquired immune responses).[33] Neither of these options has garnered sufficient support to convince the preponderance of those who study Crohn's, let alone those who suffer from it. Whether or not these competing theories ever supersede autoimmune explanations, or whether new multifactorial theories supersede immunological ones, the very notion that Crohn's ever constituted an autoimmune disease itself has some unresolved issues. Indeed, the very notion of autoimmunity consistently creates conundrums for bioscience since it disturbs immunology's dominant dogma, which holds that the immune system exists in order to discriminate between self and not-self—where *not-self* represents not just the self's logical or *bio-logical* negation but also its enemy.

The impetus for this modern immunological paradigm derives from Australian Nobel laureate Frank Macfarlane Burnet's clonal selection theory, first proposed in 1957. This theory posited "self/not-self discrimination" as both the theoretical and the evolutionary crux of immune function.[34] Rather than simply accept the then-prevailing premise that immune function defends the organism from threatening foreign entities (primarily bacterial, viral, and fungal), Burnet asked how an organism identifies foreignness in the first place. He proposed that this distinction depends on a logically and bio-logically prior difference between self and not-self. This bio-logical opposition in turn explained why, under normal (i.e., not pathological) circumstances, the components of our immune systems do not react with, let alone act against, our own body's constituents. He called this fundamental phenomenon "immunological tolerance." In Burnet's estimation, the immunological self remains "the same as" itself only insofar as it does not respond to or react against itself during the course of our lives. That is, we maintain ourselves as selves by immunologically tolerating "self"; conversely, whatever the immune system tolerates counts as self.

Autoimmunity calls this basic premise into question. It suggests that our immunological self can sometimes appear to itself as other than itself—if not as its own worst enemy—thereby muddying the clear opposition between self and not-self. In other words, autoimmunity is an event in which the immunological self cannot tolerate parts of itself.[35] Or, as my doctors metaphorically conveyed this concept to me, in which you are allergic to yourself, rejecting yourself, or eating yourself alive. More than a century ago, long before immunology understood much about how immunity worked, Paul Ehrlich, one of immunity's first theorists and a corecipient of the 1908 Nobel Prize in medicine along with Élie Metchnikoff (whose work I discuss later), found the possibility of such self-reactivity so absurd that he referred to it as the *"horror autotoxicus."*[36] In his estimation, the notion that an organism might do itself harm (or be its own enemy) was too horrible to even consider. Alas, some of us live with that horror, and some die from it as well—which is why it might also be worth considering the complicated contexts within which one's life becomes a horror and, thereby, a precipitating autoimmune factor.

According to immunological doctrine, autoimmunity should not logically—or indeed *bio*-logically—exist. Yet unfortunately it seems to, and there's the rub. According to current biomedical estimates, between sixty and eighty diseases and conditions are considered to have autoimmune etiologies, including, in addition to Crohn's disease: type 1 diabetes, multiple sclerosis, myasthenia gravis, lupus erythematosus, ankylosing spondylitis, ulcerative colitis, rheumatoid arthritis, alopecia, Addison's disease, Graves' disease, Hashimoto's disease, scleroderma, and Guillain-Barré syndrome, among many others; more continue to be added to the list on a regular basis. In light of these proliferating autoimmune complications, in which self and not-self seem to fold back onto one another—and hence defy the assumed differences between them—bioscience has had to work hard to maintain its faith in Burnet's basic split. In the face of the increasing empirical evidence that the self/not-self distinction does not always hold true—which may also indicate that the law of noncontradiction that underwrites scientific rationality doesn't always apply to living organisms—medicine has had to construct an array of complex theories to explain the expanding autoimmune enigma. Thus far, however, none of them can resolve the persistent paradoxes that autoimmunity introduces, and so autoimmunity remains an immunological impasse.[37]

Whether or not its precipitating impulses are autoimmune, immunodeficient, autoinflammatory, or some other etiology altogether, no consensus exists about how Crohn's occurs, let alone why it occurs, when it occurs, to those of us in whom it occurs.[38] Given such persistent uncertainties, it seems less surprising that there are still no treatments that address whatever provokes it. Instead, because its inflaming factors remain elusive, the therapeutic strategies today remain much the same as they were four decades ago when I first encountered them: that is, suppress the symptoms by disrupting the deleterious immune developments that seem to provoke them. Needless to say, symptom suppression through immune modulation requires rolling out some heavy artillery. (One review of this kind of treatment calls it "the sledgehammer of immunosuppression."[39]) Therefore, immediately after my diagnosis, this medical mobilization moved my life into an acute pharmacological phase. My doctors prescribed massive doses of prednisone, still one of the most popular and powerful glucocorticoid medications, to subdue the inflammation that had seared the surface of my small bowel.[40] I don't remember that there was much discussion about prednisone at the time: about how or why it worked, about its short- or long-term side effects, about how it might affect my moods or my energy, let alone about how it might impact the processes of puberty (which of course it does—it's a cortisone steroid). Instead, what I do remember are the little Dixie cups filled with bitter white tablets that I would gulp down and follow by a Maalox chaser chugged straight from the bottle to shield my mucus membranes from the pills' toxic tendencies. By definition, all effective pharmaceuticals have some degree of toxicity, which is what makes them pharmaceuticals to begin with. The ancient Greeks already knew this, which is why their word *pharmakon*, from which all our various *pharma-* words derive, carried two antithetical meanings: remedy and poison—along with a third inflection, scapegoat.[41] This derivation reminds us that if something has the power to help us, it probably also has the power to do harm and also to take the blame for it—an insight we are well advised to recall, and not just when it involves medicine.

Although prednisone remains a staple immunosuppressant, routinely deployed for all kinds of acute inflammations, the Crohn's pharmacopoeia has expanded significantly in the decades since my diagnosis. Today it includes a range of so-called biologic drugs—the previously mentioned monoclonal antibodies that disrupt the actions of tumor necrosis factor alpha and interleukin-17A, key agents in immune function and apparently also in immune dysfunction—as well as other more or less toxic chemotherapies. Forty years ago, however, none of these treatments existed, so I consumed mass quantities of prednisone for more than ten years. Given the newer options and prednisone's serious side effects, I doubt that anyone, and especially not an adolescent, would still be subjected to such a sustained regime of corticosteroids. Back then there wasn't much choice, or much general information, so despite the fact that it produced numerous harmful consequences, there wasn't much discussion about them. Even when we did suspect that something might be amiss, my doctor dramatically downplayed it. For example, I remember that my mother once asked my gastroenterologist why, after taking prednisone for over a year, I weighed a hundred pounds more than when I started. He replied, with no apparent irony or concern, "Oh, well, he's just big boned." (I kid you not—and by the way, I'm not.)

Today, if you look up prednisone on a website like Drugs.com, you can immediately discover a panoply of potential problems, including (in alphabetical order): aggression; agitation; anxiety; blurred vision; decrease in the amount of urine; dizziness; fast, slow, pounding, or irregular heartbeat or pulse; headache; irritability; mental depression; mood changes; nervousness; noisy, rattling breathing; numbness or tingling in the arms or legs; pounding in the ears; shortness of breath; swelling of the fingers, hands, feet, or lower legs; trouble thinking, speaking, or walking; troubled breathing at rest; weight gain—not to mention a cornucopia of long-term metabolic, cardiovascular, endocrinological, gastrointestinal, musculoskeletal, ocular, dermatological, hematological, and psychological aftereffects. However, in the decades before the internet, when none of this information was at our fingertips, I had no inkling that any of these could occur. In addition to the weight gain (from which I still bear the stretch marks more than four decades later), I certainly had almost all of the psychological signs (again in alphabetical order: aggression, agitation, anxiety, irritability, mental depression, mood swings, and nervousness), all of which my doctors and my parents seemed to attribute to adolescence rather than to the drugs I was on. As a result, no one bothered to consider that I might benefit from any help beyond what the medicine provided.

Once I was diagnosed with Crohn's, my parents assumed medicine could and would (and should?) provide all the relevant resources to treat my problem. I had a gastrointestinal disease, and so I went to the gastroenterologist. According to the anatomical atlas that explains medical specialization, what more could I ask for? Almost by definition, anything else would have seemed excessive.[42] Hence, when I begged my father, the physical chemist who didn't believe medicine was a "real science" (which it's not), to send me to a psychotherapist, he sarcastically shot back, "You've seen too many Woody Allen movies." He always excelled at the quick, cutting zinger, a talent that I alas also inherited.

The problem with relying on medical knowledge as the main conduit to healing is twofold: not only does medicine not know everything, but it also doesn't even always tell us everything it does know. In my case, not only did I never hear that medicine doesn't know the causes of Crohn's and therefore could provide no cure, but I was never informed about the toxicity of the drugs on which I came to depend. (I only found this out a decade later when, after my small bowel resection, I was taken off them too abruptly, precipitating a world-shattering withdrawal—about which more to come in chapter 3). Just as importantly, medicine's knowledge claims can also lead us to discount the things we might intuit about our own experiences, especially those that medicine doesn't consider relevant.

I'm not suggesting that my doctors should have known that as well as manifesting biochemical and cellular disturbances to my intestinal epithelium, my symptoms also manifested more or less intelligent responses to the persistent psychological and emotional problems plaguing my life at the time—for example, going through puberty as a proto-queer kid in 1970s small-town America decades before *Will & Grace*, *Queer Eye*, *Glee*, or *Pose* appeared in our living rooms (something I myself only began to grasp after finally getting into psychotherapy in the wake of the aforementioned prednisone withdrawal). Nevertheless, given what they did know about prednisone, they probably should have recognized that anyone taking large doses of it while going through puberty and adolescence might experience emotional challenges that could have benefited from some professional recognition, if not therapeutic support.[43]

Lacking any such encouragement or insight from my doctors and given my investments in medicine as the fount of all knowledge about my illness, I discounted my experience of living with these side effects as irrelevant. As I mentioned in chapter 1, the distinction between illness (how we experience our interrupted lives) and disease (what doctors diagnose as our pathologies) only occurred to me after chatting with Dr. J. over a decade and a half later; hence, at the time I assumed these were the same things. And, if what my doctors told me about what was occurring in my body bore the scientific seal of approval (as I then believed), who was I to argue?

As a result of my blind faith in medicine, none of the meanings I attributed to my incontinence, my cramps, my weight gain, my anxieties, my mood swings, or my depression impressed me as important. Instead, I imagined that *I* was my main problem—after all, my doctors had told me I was either allergic to myself, rejecting myself, or eating myself alive—and my parents, who were equally invested in the therapeutic powers of medical knowledge, appeared to concur. What I didn't understand then, that I do now, is that medicine only became medicine in our modern scientific sense by driving a wedge between our imaginations and its knowledge. As chapter 3 underscores, this decisive distinction, imagination versus knowledge, continues to underwrite the way medicine legitimates its own relation to scientific understanding. And paradoxically, this opposition remains at the heart of the medical imagination insofar as medicine imagines itself as radically distinct from other modes of healing and especially insofar as it aspires to scientific status.

Yet the imagination is never ancillary to illness; it is the matrix within which illnesses arise insofar as illness is always a human experience. For, as Foucault succinctly reminds us, "There is no experience which is not a way of thinking."[44] In other words, illnesses do not take place only within our organs, tissues, cells, and molecules, even if diseases might. They arise within our lives, and how we make sense of them informs how we live (with) them. As Arthur Frank reminded us in chapter 1, what medicine tells us about our cellular and molecular processes describes part of the story at best. The rest depends on us.

Thus, even if medical knowledge can support and sustain us by diagnosing or treating a disease, it cannot actually know what we're going through. Nevertheless, because it presents itself to us as knowledge incarnate—and moreover because we often desire this knowing incarnation to save us—medicine can incite us to side with it and thereby to divide ourselves against ourselves. Aligning our best interests with medical diagnoses and treatments, we often ignore our own innate resources, including our powerful imaginations, which can be crucial allies for our healing. When we depend on medicine to heal us, we tend to credit its knowledge and authority rather than appreciate our own healing capacities. And since we pay (or, if we're lucky, our insurance pays) to receive medicine's insights, most of us who rely on them accept this deal as a given.

As a result, we often fail to recognize that while medicine has many amazing means of intervening on our behalf, it alone does not have the capacity to heal us. Instead, insofar as healing happens, it always happens under our own auspices. If we heal, our bodies do the healing, no matter how much support—including life support—medicine might provide. Regrettably, then, the formidable powers of modern medicine can mask the value of our own healing tendencies. Medicine might even appear to us as the source of our salvation rather than a resource that at best shores up and encourages our own intrinsic capacities. This is not to say that medical knowledge commands our complicity or our compliance; however, if we don't reflect on medicine's practices and how they came into being, we might forget that its knowledge has some very real limits and that, conversely, we are always more complicated than it knows.

As you've hopefully gleaned by now, medicine modifies us not only with its treatments but also with its ways of thinking—which are often one and the same process. As the feminist philosopher of science Isabelle Stengers acutely puts it, "Medicine cannot be reduced to a response to individual suffering, and it is not just the business of the doctor and his patient. The way in which humans hope, anticipate, fear, and imagine, the way in which they not only conceive but also construct their personal and collective identities, crucially depends on the meanings given by themselves and by others to what affects them."[45] In other words, when we accept medicine's advice, we also take in how it conceives both the vital matter that we are and the vital vulnerabilities that matter to us so long as we're alive. After all, to be alive is by definition to be vulnerable (from the Latin *vulnus*, meaning wound), which is why healing matters so much in keeping us alive.[46]

Medicine seeks to shore up our vulnerabilities by therapeutically applying its knowledge to our bodies. In some cases—but by no means all—this applied knowledge can relieve our suffering, which offers us a strong incentive to incorporate it into ourselves. Unfortunately, sometimes this incorporation encourages us to give medicine more credit than it is due. Or, more accurately, sometimes it encourages us to discredit our own insights and to adopt its understandings as the only ones that count. Because medicine prescribes thoughts along with its therapies, these thoughts can infect us both somatically and psychically.

For example, taking prednisone with breakfast every morning for over a decade did not just modulate (alas, very imperfectly) the inflammatory inclinations that troubled my guts (as well as incite the slew of physical and emotional side effects described above). It also offered a pharmaceutical communion with a biomedical faith whose autoimmune dogma informed me—via its officiants, my doctors—that I was either allergic to myself, rejecting myself, or eating myself alive. Of course, none of these metaphors actually explained the crap that was happening to me, and, unfortunately, spending years making sense of Crohn's disease in these terms did not help me get through them with much grace or ease. Yet, sadly, that's the way my doctors presented it to me, and so that's how I imagined it.

According to my gastroenterologists, Crohn's was an inflammatory bowel disease localized in my gut; therefore, it was certainly not something I was just imagining. (I was fortunate in this way. My friend Rebecca's doctors told her she was just imagining her back pain, after they failed to correctly diagnose ankylosing spondylitis and instead performed two unnecessary and debilitating spinal fusions that seriously exacerbated rather than alleviated her suffering.[47]) This declaration did prove beneficial in that no one could deny the reality of my suffering any longer, as my parents had been doing for a while. My diarrhea and weight loss were no longer (just) symptoms of excessive nervousness, nor of (just) anxiety or depression—which my Jewish family considered normal and not pathological anyway. (For example, my father often referred to me using the Yiddish equivalent of "nervous Nellie"—turning my ambient anxiety and incipient gendered sexuality into an epithet he could use to sarcastically dismiss the significance of both.) Instead, the medical confirmation of Crohn's definitively pinpointed my problem in the lining of my small intestine and thereby gave my daily dis-ease a specifically somatic focus. Yet, even in medicine's own terms, this specificity didn't really make sense: if Crohn's has an autoimmune etiology, and if the nonlocalized immune system permeates the entire organism, then Crohn's must be a full-body experience, which is certainly how it felt.

Medicine's explanations contain its concepts, and thus when we receive these explanations, especially in the form of diagnoses or prescriptions, we ingest them as well. These conceptual implications are rarely made explicit to us, but they remain forceful nonetheless. Consider one of the conceptual complications that arose during my initial diagnostic drama: when they first explained Crohn's disease to me, my doctors told me that a high proportion of those affected by Crohn's were Ashkenazi Jews. Since they couldn't provide me with any other explanation for why I'd gotten so sick, they offered this epidemiological correlation to clarify why I, in particular, was in such a shitty predicament.[48]

Now, despite being a Cohen, I had never felt particularly Jewish before. I grew up in a small town in Maryland in which there were only three Jewish families (ours, the Getzes, and the Baers), and as I mentioned earlier, my parents were devout atheists. Although we did schlep up to New York City, where my father's family lived, to celebrate Passover and Rosh Hashanah, these events did not inspire much religious affiliation in me—especially as my mother usually complained constantly about the hollowness of the occasions and spent much of the time reading from her archive of leftist and pro-Palestinian literature. Indeed, I'm sure it was more than just a random coincidence that at the age of thirteen, instead of having a bar mitzvah, I was admitted to the hospital, thereby unconsciously enacting my own secular rite of passage.

Given my resolutely nonreligious background, when my doctors explained Crohn's Jewish proclivities, it made me consider my Jewish heritage in a new way. Apparently, despite how I'd been raised to think about myself, Jewishness lived in me as a hereditary fault, the genetic predisposition to suffering shitstorms betraying a legacy from ancestors with whom I otherwise felt little direct connection. My diagnosis appeared to belie my tenuous Jewish identification and instead revealed Jewishness to me as a palpable and inescapable biomolecular trace. At the time, I probably understood the Darwinian roots of contemporary genetics much as any thirteen-year-old would, that is, imperfectly. I certainly had no idea that the biological concept of heredity, of which the gene represents a material unit, was invented by Charles Darwin in *On the Origin of Species* (1859) in order to supersede Jean-Baptiste Lamarck's earlier notion that acquired traits could be "conserved" from one generation to the next. Nor would I have had a clue that Darwin, who inherited so much money that he never had to hold a job (and who, as mentioned above, some now conjecture also suffered with Crohn's), had metaphorically derived the biological notion of heredity from the ancient legal transfer of property after death, from which he himself had so greatly benefited. Although Darwin did not have a genetic understanding of biological inheritance (since genes did not get named as units of heredity until 1909), he nevertheless reinterpreted the living organism as a kind of heritable property, an interpretation consonant with the prevailing legal and political perspectives on personhood at the time.

Because I lacked any awareness of heredity's genealogy, the inference that I drew from my doctors' remarks concerning Crohn's Jewish propensities precipitated a somewhat distorted self-image. Until then I may have had a vague sense that my personal peculiarities had strong links to my parents' and grandparents' dispositions, for example, believing that my digestive disorder was somehow "like" my grandmother's persistent pancreatitis, which is how my relatives accounted for it until I was officially diagnosed. (Behind her back, they also attributed my grandmother's intestinal complaints to her excessive-if-not-hypochondriacal anxiety and depression, traits I probably also shared.) Yet the notion that I had inherited a disposition or proclivity to digestive distemper through a quasi-racial-cultural-religious lineage revised my sense of how deeply Jewishness and its genetic past lived in me. Therefore, when my doctors alerted me to my (supposed) hereditary tendency to Crohn's, they revealed me to myself in a new way. If, on the one hand, I now believed that something was wrong in me, as clinical medicine prescribed, on the other hand, I now imagined that this fault had been genetically scripted at some obscure point in the Jewish past, long before I'd even been conceived. From this contradictory set of ideas, I concluded that Crohn's proved that I was both fated to be defective and the source of my own suffering—no doubt a very anxious and very Jewish double whammy. (And if you haven't figured it out by now, Burrill Crohn and Henry Janowitz were Jewish too.)

This is not to say that medicine led me to conjure this imaginary solution to its conceptual impasse; however, it did overtly and covertly offer its concepts as tools for making sense of what was happening. These concepts in turn prompted me to imagine certain—perhaps untenable—connections between what was going on in my gut and what was going on in my head. (Today's acceptance of the enteric nervous system and the "gut-brain-microbiome axis" as robust biomedical concepts might make such familiar conjectures seem more valid.) I confess that I have a very vivid imagination, so the ways my doctors represented my problem to me may have unduly shaped the terms within which I attempted to contain the uncontainable shit that Crohn's stirred up. Be that as it may, the mental perceptions catalyzed by medical concepts convey more connotations than medicine alone can know. Medicine's concepts may not intend to do so. After all, they simply claim to represent the best attempts to grasp the physiological processes through which diseases transpire in order to redirect them toward therapeutic ends. Yet they nevertheless also imaginatively inform the lived experiences of those of us who naively trust the "truth" of medicine's dictums.

In the decade between my initial diagnosis and my radical recovery from near-death, the medical interpretations of my illness confounded me. Believing that I suffered from an autoimmune disease challenged my ability to make sense not only of who I was, or of what was happening to me, but also of what my "self" meant, especially insofar as I was apparently allergic to mine. Needless to say, lots of young people flounder in similar waters; I suppose such floundering features prominently in many an adolescence and early adulthood. However, because mine was an adolescence on steroids, it proved especially difficult to swim athwart the conceptual undertow. The ideas that doctors planted in my imagination flourished, no doubt fertilized by all the prednisone they prescribed. Imagining my self as the enemy of myself—or indeed imagining my self as my enemy, trying to grapple with the implication that I was both the cause and the effect of my suffering, or turning over and over the ways my body had supposedly turned upon itself, provided little help in understanding how to live a healthy life with Crohn's. In fact, at the time, the possibility of living a healthy, let alone happy, life with Crohn's entirely eluded my imagination—and apparently my doctors' as well, since they never mentioned it. Instead, thinking Crohn's was my shitty lot in life led me to believe that my self was irreparably shitty. I had no idea how to resolve this dilemma, and so I resigned myself to living a crappy life with a crappy self. (You can see why I begged my father to send me to a therapist and why his snarky put-down remains so memorable.)

Adolescence on steroids is a bit like having a medically induced mental illness. Not that anyone seemed to notice this then, but maybe that's because adolescence seems like a mental illness to many adults. Perhaps, if the predni-sone had stopped the debilitating diarrhea, it wouldn't have been quite so bad. But it didn't, and so, between the ages of thirteen and twenty-three, my life was entirely circumscribed by experiences of Crohn's, many involving incontinence. Not surprisingly, incontinence requires a lot of careful planning and excessive vigilance, for example: always sitting at the end of the aisle, intuiting the loca-tion of the nearest toilet, carrying several extra pairs of underwear, dreading any confined space where I couldn't immediately escape to relieve my bowels—all this became second nature, as did the wracking cramps, the gaseous explo-sions, the nausea and vomiting, and the anal abrasions. (You wouldn't believe how harsh the toilet paper in public bathrooms, gas stations, and outhouses can be or what it can do to sensitive mucus membranes.)

Then there were the joys of attending a large public high school with thirty-six hundred teens, where the partitions between the stalls in the boys' toilets had been removed to discourage loitering and smoking. I used to take massive doses of vitamin C and give myself an enema every morning before school in the hope that by preemptively purging my bowels I could avoid having to expose myself to the taunting and humiliation that my effusive excretions elicited from the boys who always lingered in the bathroom rather than go to class. Unfortunately, these strategies never actually preempted anything. To my great relief, after a year of such indignities, the school nurse took pity on me and al-lowed me to use the special toilet reserved for menstruating girls. This was an incredible boon, even though for many of my peers it simply confirmed my already well-established reputation as a fag. (On the positive side, however, the injustice of having to wait for the school's one private toilet along with girls having their periods made my commitment to feminism—passed down from my mother—much more visceral.) All that, plus the extra hundred pounds of fat, the moon face, the excessive acne, and the maddening mood swings, made each day of high school a joy to wake up to. I'm joking of course—it was not fun. And although the social stigma abated considerably after high school, the shit didn't. It just continued, getting episodically worse in college and then per-sistently worse in my first two years of graduate school. At that point, I had no idea how it might ever get better. Apparently, neither did my doctors.

If you have a chronic illness, dealing with doctors is part of the routine. Because I was on high doses of steroids, plus a few other meds to deal with cramps, nausea, pain, and so on, I would have to visit my gastroenterologist in his dingy office in downtown Baltimore every six to eight weeks. During high school, my mother drove us the thirty-five miles or so from our small town in northern Maryland to Baltimore; during college, I took the train from Washington, DC, and my mother picked me up at the Amtrak station near Dr. D.'s office. During these eight years, my relationship with my doctor was entirely triangulated through my relationship with my mother. If you think Oedipal triangles are tricky, try medical ones—sadly, I had both. I was so entangled in this triangle of care, knowledge, and drugs that I only applied to two colleges and chose Georgetown because it allowed me to keep Dr. D. as my physician, despite the fact that it was a Jesuit university and I was a proto-queer-commie Jew. This was probably not the wisest decision. You could say my relationship with Dr. D. was overdetermined. Of course, he did prescribe powerful and addictive drugs to me (without ever informing me about their side effects). He also described these drugs as the only prescriptions on offer to stanch the deluge of diarrhea that defined my daily life. Since I had no other ways to try to modulate the river of shit that swept through me—sweeping me along with it—not surprisingly, I believed I needed him as my life preserver. Unfortunately, I really didn't like him.

Dr. D. came into my life after my pediatrician sent me to the internist who sent me to the head of gastroenterology at Johns Hopkins. This "world-famous" gastroenterologist then palmed me off on one of his former residents, Dr. D., who now trained other doctors at the nearby University of Maryland hospital. Doctor D. had no bedside manner to speak of. English was his third language, so communication was stilted at best. Also, he had terrible touch. One of the key moments in any gastroenterological exam involves palpating the abdomen. In our current age of high-tech, computer-driven, corporate health care, it's probably one of the few medical procedures that still requires a doctor to regularly touch a patient in order to treat them. In Dr. D.'s cramped little exam room, I'd lie back on the table and then lift up my shirt and stare at the sad spider plant hanging above me as he'd press on my viscera chanting the gastroenterologists' mantra: "Does this hurt? Does this hurt?" Not surprisingly, this form of interaction is neither relaxing nor reassuring. Between the drugs, the exams, his general lack of interpersonal connection, and the fact that none of these significantly interrupted my incontinence, visits to Dr. D. did not lift my spirits. Nor did they help me believe that an alternative life was possible.

This was not surprising because, in addition to the powerful drugs, the painful palpations, and the depressing office, Dr. D. imbued me with a form of thinking—through both his descriptions and his prescriptions—that radically limited how I imagined my illness. If we recall Foucault's admonition, "there is no experience which is not a way of thinking"—or consider Alfred North Whitehead's assessment that "the quality of an act of experience is largely determined by the factor of thinking which it contains"[49]—then because my relations with Dr. D. saturated how I thought about Crohn's, they also saturated how I experienced it as well. And as for the quality of that experience . . . well, let's just say I don't recommend it. While Dr. D.'s care no doubt staved off the worst consequences of Crohn's for a while, it didn't exactly make me better and certainly not healthier. Under this regime I endured the double indignities of Crohn's and prednisone for more than a decade. There were ups and downs, but the general drift was downward, since the inflammation never entirely abated. In fact, over time my symptoms just got increasingly insistent.

Fortunately, by the time the shit really started hitting the fan, I had moved on from Dr. D. to Dr. B. This move coincided with my move from Georgetown to Stanford when I began my PhD program there. One of the great things about getting my PhD at Stanford, over and above the excellent education in the California country-club environment (where Rodin sculptures and exotic fruit trees dotted the campus), was the incredible student health plan that afforded me access to one of the world's best—that is, most expensive and well-endowed— hospitals. When I arrived with my entire medical portfolio, I went straight to the student health office, which promptly outsourced me to a gastroenterologist affiliated with Stanford's medical complex. Dr. B.'s office provided a study in contrasts with Dr. D.'s. No dowdy brick office building in downtown Baltimore this time; rather, a modern, light-filled, glass-and-steel structure in Palo Alto, filled with a profusion of vibrant plants, modern furniture, and white-coated medical professionals bustling about. If only because Dr. B.'s realm in the GI department radiated a state-of-the-art aesthetic, it immediately inspired more confidence in medicine than I'd ever had before.

This is not to say that Dr. B.'s treatment plan differed much from Dr. D.'s. Palpation, prednisone, and persistent intestinal pain still ruled the day. But Dr. B. had a pleasant personality; he could even joke with me about the indignities of incontinence. Even better, he treated me as an adult, which Dr. D. never had— in part because I met him when I was thirteen and in part because my mother always mediated my relationship with him—and Dr. B. even considered my ideas about my treatment relevant information. Of course, by the time I met him, I did have extensive experience with Crohn's and hence had some insight into what worked and what didn't. So, although not exactly acknowledging me as a fellow expert in the field, at least he recognized me as a well-informed participant. This is not to say ours was a perfect partnership because the same limits to medical knowing still applied. Like all my doctors before him, Dr. B. never said he didn't know why Crohn's occurred or how it could be cured, nor did he mention the side effects of the prednisone, doses of which escalated throughout my time under his care. And, of course, he never uttered the word *healing* in my presence or suggested I check out any other nonmedical forms of therapeutic intervention that flourished in the Bay Area (e.g., psychotherapy or any of the somatic modalities the rest of this book describes). Still, liking one's doctor does have benefits.

Needless to say, given all the unknowns that still hover around Crohn's, no one knows why my symptoms got progressively more acute during my first two years in graduate school—though after much reflection, I have some suspicions. As the milligrams of prednisone ratcheted up, my moon face blossomed. I dragged myself from class to class, extra underwear at the ready, toting my heating pad with me, which I'd plug in and strap on as soon as I sat down at the seminar table. I can't remember exactly what tests I underwent at this point because all the barium swallows and enemas have blurred together over the years, but I have no doubt that there were a few. At the very least there must have been a lot of blood work because whenever the doses of prednisone increased, there was always more blood work. Yet, despite the daily demands of defecation and the steroid-induced insanity, I tried to live my life on drugs as best a twenty-two-year-old could. Because it was Northern California in the early 1980s, that involved a lot of dancing, the Grateful Dead, and other more uplifting drugs.

Out of this heady mix, I accidentally discovered that marijuana not only got me high but also relieved my cramping and intestinal spasms. Decades before the phrase "medical marijuana" ever tripped off anyone's tongue, I had no idea that marijuana could do such a thing, or I would have become a pothead much sooner. (My friend Julie was luckier. Her gastroenterologist, who must have been way cooler than Dr. D., clued her into this possibility in high school.) In many ways, smoking marijuana was my first intimation that nonmedical remedies had much to offer. Today I'd call marijuana a "teacher plant" whose vibrant *viriditas* leaps out at anyone who's ever watched it grow. The plant practically eats light, transforming the carbon dioxide it absorbs from the air and the nutrients and water it takes up through its roots into complex biochemicals which, when appropriately treated, release organic molecules into the bloodstream that attach to endogenous cannabinoid receptors found not only in our brains but also in our guts. (Remember, the gut has most of the same neuroreceptors as the brain.) In fact, marijuana acts as a smooth muscle relaxant in general, which is why it's also helpful for menstruation and childbirth. A friend who had three children at home told me each time she went into labor she rolled a pin joint, and it really took the edge off the experience. Why humans evolved neuroreceptors that resonate with marijuana's analgesic powers remains a mystery.[50] Nevertheless, empirically speaking, it works. And because Stanford was just a hop, skip, and a jump from the mecca of marijuana cultivation in Northern California, I had easy access to some of the best *viriditas* available. After my initial discovery, I quickly became a connoisseur, and it totally changed my relation to Crohn's by relaxing my relation to my gut.

Fortunately for me—although it definitely didn't seem that way at the time—my California lifestyle didn't involve a lot of sex. Prednisone put a damper on that, as did the debilitating diarrhea. It's hard to imagine sexual intimacy with someone when you might shit yourself at any moment. Turns out that might have been a lucky miss, since this was exactly the time when HIV/AIDS (which hadn't yet been named as such) began to make its appearance among gay men of my age, and San Francisco was one of its epicenters. Indeed, my best medical one-liner of all time resulted from this historical and geographical coincidence. In the weeks before my devastating bleed-out, I underwent a barrage of tests and consultations. One day the infectious diseases team showed up in my room in the Hoover Pavilion. They told me that they had begun to see a number of gay men who were manifesting debilitating (fortunately they didn't say deadly) clusters of symptoms, some of which seemed similar to mine. They told me they didn't know what caused it, but they used the term GRID—gay-related immune deficiency—and they hypothesized that it might be sexually transmitted.[51] Then they asked me if I thought I might have it. Without thinking, I quipped, "Not unless you believe in immaculate infection." Then we all laughed uproariously. It remains the best medical laugh of my life. As it turns out, because the first blood test for HIV (called HTLV-III at the time) didn't appear until 1984, the massive number of blood transfusions I received in the hospital constituted my greatest risk for exposure to HIV.

Since chapter 1 began by recounting the exciting events that culminated in my sojourn in the Hoover Pavilion, I won't dwell on the remainder of my acute decline. I want this book to focus on healing, not illness—even if the latter did precipitate my awareness of the former. So, let me wrap up this sickly part of my tale by reminding you of what I learned the hard way from my first ten years of living with Crohn's. On the one hand, I learned that medicine has some very powerful resources. When you're critically or acutely ill, don't hesitate to get yourself to a doctor. They might have treatments to offer that can assuage, if not cure, what ails you. On the other hand, it slowly dawned on me that when taking in medicine's treatments, we also take in certain ways of thinking about ourselves that might not fully appreciate our own innate reparative capacities as living organisms. Since its inception, medicine has staked its claims to therapeutic superiority on its knowing abilities. From the introduction of diagnosis and prognosis in ancient Greece to our current investments in high-tech interventions and evidence-based medicine, knowledge has always constituted medicine's bailiwick. Yet as powerful as medicine's knowing ways often prove to be, like any knowledge practice, they always have their limits—even if our physicians don't always know or say what those might be.

If medicine has always predicated its authority to govern our lives on such knowledge claims, it has also assumed that this knowledge alone provides the best basis for therapy. Thus, it does not always recognize that we are more than it—and we—can know. This "more than" does not undercut what can be known but instead reframes it, resituating knowing within living, where it has always resided anyway (as Bergson and Canguilhem reminded us). Living might include knowing as one of its vital assets, as one of the ways life extends itself in time and space. Yet, beyond the knowable or the calculable lies the improbable, which may or may not always happen but nevertheless might merit our attention and esteem. Healing is one of these incalculable tendencies, and we all owe our lives to it, some of us more than others. Unfortunately, as the agency of bioscience and biotech have captured more and more of our interest and our desire over the past century and a half, the apparent value of healing in medicine has waned. When we seek medical treatments—if we can afford them and if they are available, which in the race- and class-stratified United States is not at all guaranteed—we often imagine the clinic as the epicenter of therapeutic influence. Sometimes this turns out to be the case, however not always.[52] And quite often, when it comes to chronic illnesses, perhaps less often than we might like.

## THREE

## We Are More Imaginative Than We Think

The body itself simply from the laws of its own nature, can do many things
which its mind wonders at.—SPINOZA, *Ethics*, III p2 Schol. (1667)

Leaving the hospital after my prolonged sojourn evoked all the joys of any liber-
ation. While I was certainly grateful to be alive, and appreciated how much the
physicians, nurses, and other hospital workers had contributed to my going-on-
living, a hospital is not a very convivial context. It can do a lot to keep us alive
when things get critical, but healing does not figure prominently in its mission
either medically or financially—let alone aesthetically. In the hospital, most
of the patterns of daily life that make us feel at home in the world get stripped
down to their essential minimum: life support. Hospital food serves as a widely
recognized index for this minimalist ethos. And in the days before laptops, cell
phones, and the internet, hospitalization induced a fair amount of isolation.
Despite visits from friends, landline phone calls placed through the hospital
switchboard, and lots of reading material (including Foucault of course), my
hospital stay proved a rather long slog. Thus, returning to the shabby Eichler
house in Palo Alto that I shared with four other grad students, I felt restored to
the land of milk and honey (which, given the current value of that classic mid-
century-modern California vernacular house in Silicon Valley, perhaps it was).

I didn't necessarily go around singing the "L'chaim" song from *Fiddler on the Roof*, but there was undoubtedly an initial spring in my step. Alas, that upbeat feeling didn't last long.

Needless to say, such transitions are bound to be arduous and, hence, benefit from expenditures of energy and resources—if they're available, it really helps. One of the many problems with American health care is that once you leave the hospital (if you even get to stay, since many procedures, including major surgeries, are now performed on an outpatient basis), you're mostly on your own. It's then up to you and those around you to pick up the slack. Much of this responsibility falls on friends and families. If you're single and alone, good luck to you. Fortunately, although I was definitely single, I had both friends and family, and they helped smooth my passage. For example, my parents, who had rarely bought me presents as a child—instead reminding me that everything I wanted was a capitalist ploy (which it was)—bought me a car. A stripped-down, bottom-of-the-line Ford Escort, but a car, nonetheless.

They also agreed to pay for psychotherapy—despite my having seen even more Woody Allen movies—to help me reorient myself in my new body, now missing a substantial portion of my small intestine, as well as more than a few bits and pieces of my liver. I clearly needed some help sorting out a new self-image. For example, was the major scar that ran down the middle of my abdomen and then curved around my belly button, forming a giant upside-down question mark, ironic, or weirdly appropriate, or both? My body had definitely changed, so I needed to update my ways of thinking about it. No doubt, my parents' unprecedented generosity—rooted in their middle-class financial security, which was in turn deeply planted in their politically committed, Jewish-inflected, Depression-era abstemiousness—was certainly very lucky for me because it soon became clear that even though I was getting stronger physically and my scars were gradually becoming less monstrous and more familiar, something was not only psychically off-kilter, it was getting progressively worse.

While at this point in my life I could discuss the physical manifestations of Crohn's in exquisite detail, I didn't have a clue about how to recognize, let alone convey, its psychological implications. If it didn't exude from my ass, I had no idea how to represent the shit that was happening to me. Moreover, I had no idea about how to address it or to whom to address it. After all, why would I tell a gut doctor that a hollowness had erupted at the center of my existence and that, like an emotional black hole, it had begun to suck away all my newfound vitality? That fall semester I remember going through the routine of my normal life as a graduate student: reading books, writing papers, listening to music, getting stoned, going dancing, even as these things started to seem as if they occurred on the far side of an unbreakable sheet of ice. I felt frozen, deeply, at some essential if not exactly physical level. Everything in me seemed voided and devoid, cold to the touch, inert, dead—although I knew I wasn't really dead because I had just survived my death. When I tried to explain this to one of my roommates one night (no doubt while we were stoned), she freaked out and told me she couldn't deal with me anymore and that I should get myself to a therapist. That turned out to be excellent advice.

One of my other roommates, who had recently begun exploring her sexual desires for other women, had a therapist a short bike ride way, so I made an appointment with her. At the time, Joann was a lesbian goddess. She'd just written a popular book about lesbian sex and how to survive "lesbian bed death" and even appeared on *Oprah* during the short time I was seeing her. (One day my mother called me up to tell me that she'd just watched *Oprah* and my therapist was on discussing how to improve lesbian sex life.) In many ways, Joann was completely the wrong therapist for me—except, after five minutes she turned out to be the best therapist I could have picked. Meeting her was kismet. Walking into her latter-day lesbian-feminist hippie pad in downtown Palo Alto (she had been a Stanford undergraduate in the late '60s, so she came by it honestly) completely changed my life, if only because she clued me into something none of my doctors had bothered to mention. A few minutes after I started telling Joann about what was going on with me, she put up her hand and said, "Stop. You are having prednisone withdrawal."

Someone who has been taking high doses of prednisone for very long periods of time and stops too quickly (before their adrenal glands have a chance to kick back into gear) can experience intense psychological reactions, including psychosis and dissociation, she explained. I wasn't psychotic, but I was entirely dissociated—although I had no idea what that meant at the time. You can find out about prednisone withdrawal quite easily online these days; however, in the pre-internet, pre–informational packaging, pre-web-based-illness-support-community era, such esoteric knowledge remained sequestered in the hard copies of journals, hidden in medical school libraries. I was benefiting from her experience: she said, "My sister has Crohn's, and she went through the same thing. You should make an appointment with the doctor she's seeing who specializes in helping people with cancers and chronic illnesses. It might take a little while to schedule something with her, so I can work with you until then." I am forever grateful to Joann for her life-transforming interventions: first for naming my experience as (at least partly) drug induced and second for introducing me to her sister's doctor, Naomi Remen.

Naomi now goes by Rachel Remen, the name under which she has published two best-selling books, *Kitchen Table Wisdom* and *My Grandfather's Blessings*, and has become recognized as "a leading figure in body-mind medicine" (as Charlie Rose sententiously intoned before interviewing her on his TV show[1]). Part of her reputation derives from a course she designed at UCSF School of Medicine, the Healer's Art, that is now taught at more than seventy major medical schools around the world.[2] However, our time together preceded her renown. Then she was a forty-something renegade doctor, former biker, and jewelry designer who had recently given up her position as a pediatric endocrinologist at Stanford University Hospital to start a private practice counseling people with serious illnesses as well as "recovering physicians" (as she identified herself). She had also cofounded Commonweal, a comprehensive cancer care program in Bolinas, California (featured in Bill Moyers's PBS series *Healing and the Mind*[3]). Perhaps, just as importantly for this story, she had lived with Crohn's disease for almost thirty years. And because she had been diagnosed more than two decades before I embarked on my own Crohn's comedy—at a time when the treatments were much more dangerous and debilitating—her healing journey entailed more surgeries and invasive and painful treatments than mine. So I felt sure that she would understand what I was going through.

For our first session I drove my new Ford Escort up Highway 280, the "world's most beautiful highway," to meet Naomi. Winding my way along the Crystal Lakes that stretch beneath the Santa Cruz Mountains (which always reminded me I was driving through the rift valley of the San Andreas Fault *that could break open at any moment!*), it seemed as if I was moving through an allegory. This suspicion became even more intense when I traversed, first Golden Gate Park, then the Golden Gate Bridge, up over the rise of the Marin headlands, down the steep incline toward the Sausalito harbor, before exiting and parking at the marina. Walking toward the houseboat where Naomi practiced, crossing the gangplank from the pier onto the *Omphale* (which means the navel, a name conferred by a previous owner, the Western Buddhist teacher Alan Watts) only increased my allegorical suspicions. Hence, when Naomi appeared at the top of the stairs to invite me into her office, her close-cropped gray hair set aglow by light streaming from an oculus above her, the allegory seemed not just fulfilled but palpable.

To say something is allegorical doesn't mean it didn't happen. It just means that you need to think about what's happening on many levels at once to make sense of what you're dealing with and what has been dealt to you. Allegorical thinking asks you to appreciate that things are always more than they seem and certainly more than you think. Allegory teaches you to consider that the extraordinary can live within the ordinary, that the everyday is entangled with the mysterious in more ways than we usually imagine. Because I was a dogmatic materialist at the time, none of this had ever occurred to me before. Indeed, I would start to perceive these plural possibilities only after Naomi sagely reminded me, much later, that perhaps the world is not only more than it seems—a truism I'd been taught to think of as the dichotomy between appearance and reality lying at the heart of Western rationality. It might also be more creative than we think. And if so, because I am part of that world, therefore so am I. Logically that was hard to refute. Furthermore, this idea seemed to speak to all the unknown experiences I'd recently gone through and maybe even the new ones I was now going through—despite the fact that it overloaded many of the synaptic connections I'd assiduously constructed in my life heretofore.

Naomi's office was compact and well contained, as an office on a ship should be, with a porthole in one side and a wide window overlooking the bay toward the nearby Tiburon Peninsula on the other. Built-in bookshelves under the window were filled with the *Collected Works* of Carl Jung (more allegory). Two spare but comfortable chairs faced each other; there was a small desk but no other furniture. Sessions with Naomi were unbounded in time. This was not your typical "fifty minutes is an hour" therapy session. Our conversations would last several hours, though between the second and third hours they would usually wind down. I call them conversations in the strongest sense of that word because etymologically *converse* means "to turn with" (its Latin root *verso* signifies to turn often, keep turning, turn over, whirl about). When we converse deeply—and perhaps in order to converse deeply—we risk being overturned by the interaction. We risk dizziness, vertigo, and nausea in order to get a new perspective on the world.[4]

Our first conversation did just that; it turned my world upside down. After I started to fill Naomi in on the immediate backstory, recounting the tale of how I'd found my way to her, she seemed to be getting angry. Then she quietly said, "Just a minute," picked up her phone, and called my gastroenterologist. Perhaps because she had been on the faculty at Stanford Hospital for many years, she knew just how to navigate the various switchboards to get Dr. B. on the line. When she did, she began to remonstrate with him sharply (I was tempted to write "yell at," but yelling wasn't Naomi's style), emphasizing that she couldn't believe he had released me from the hospital, and even done follow-up care, yet had never mentioned that I might crash emotionally and psychologically while recovering from my treatments and simultaneously withdrawing from prednisone. Although reading Foucault's *Birth of the Clinic* in my hospital bed had provided me with the intellectual basis for conceiving a new way of thinking about medicine, Naomi's intervention completely up-ended my entire attitude toward medical care. Never before had someone with medical authority—and Naomi clearly marshaled all her Ivy-educated, Stanford-earned institutional legitimacy for that phone call—informed one of my doctors that he clearly didn't know how to take care of me. In that moment I realized that medical treatment, even treatment that saves your life, isn't always care-full and that, when it comes to healing—rather than curing—care is of the essence. That was the first hour.

The second hour moved on to my near-death experience, the trances, my surgeon's comments during our exit interview about how sick I'd been, his ad-mission that he didn't know how I'd gotten better so quickly, and the fact that the entire journey had decimated my habitual ways of knowing. Naomi gave me not just a new way to consider my experience, but a medically and person-ally informed one at that. She explained that she came from a medical family, that many of her male relatives were physicians, that her mother had been a public health nurse, and that from an early age she had known that she too would become a doctor. Much of her upbringing, as well as her subsequent medical training, had encouraged her to believe that scientific facts should provide the basis for how we know the world, including the bodies through which we live. These facts proved incredibly powerful resources, she said, and in her identification as a doctor she had ardently held onto a belief in scientific knowledge's exclusive authority—until the circumstances of her life as a patient as well as a doctor proved it untenable. She began to wonder if serious illnesses don't present us with mysteries about which, although we may come to know some things, some things will necessarily remain unknown. Even if how and why we fall ill, and how and why we recover, eventually submit to biochemical de-scriptions, what they mean for our lives may resist such reductive explanation (in both the scientific and colloquial senses). This mysteriousness probably always applies, although I now think that it's especially true for chronic illnesses like can-cers and autoimmune diseases: they confound the prevailing medical paradigms, and nobody knows why they happen, when they happen, to whom they happen.

In any case, as she listened to my story, Naomi quickly identified how incredi-bly anxious not knowing what had happened—let alone what was happening—made me, and she helped me to acknowledge it. I suppose that given my cultural inheritance as the oldest child of a physical chemist and a passionate Communist, compounded by the intellectual, professional, and personal in-vestments in knowledge acquisition demanded by my extensive education, it wasn't too hard to see that my know-it-all tendencies might be getting the better of me. Thus, her intervention turned my thinking upside down. Perhaps, she suggested, it wasn't just not knowing what I had experienced that motivated the anxious undertow which threatened to pull me under. Maybe the container I was using to hold my experiences—to make sense of my senses—was simply too small; perhaps I was trying to cram the vastness of my self into the prison-house of scientific fact.[5] Perhaps the things that had happened required me to imagine my story in a more expansive way in order to encompass all the facts in evidence. Or, to paraphrase the American philosopher William James, Naomi counseled: Nothing but experience, but all of experience.

While my reductive worldview was woven from a skein of knowledge practices largely inherited from my family, my teachers, and my culture, my ideas about living with Crohn's—both what it entailed physiologically and what it meant psychologically—came to me from my doctors. Trained in the scientific protocols that have come to define proper medical practice, they inculcated me with their explanatory habits. Accordingly, I learned that all biological phenomena, including those taking place in my gut, derived from underlying biochemical and cellular activities. Apparently no other explanations were deemed necessary. But how had medicine arrived at this parsimonious epistemological presumption? And why was it so committed to this pared-down perspective? Moreover, how did its adherence to scientific methods for knowing that arose in the seventeenth and eighteenth centuries come to control contemporary clinical practice? How did the evidence that now underwrites evidence-based medicine come to appear so self-evident that it can readily discount healing experiences like mine? And why do these authorized ways of knowing disqualify such healing experiences despite the fact that so many of them happen?

In our era, biomedicine (i.e., medicine that bases its treatments on biological and biochemical experimentation and analysis) dominates the therapeutic marketplace; however, this dominance didn't yet prevail at the turn of the twentieth century.[6] The sociologist Paul Starr has wonderfully narrated the story of medicine's "social transformation" in North America, identifying the period between 1850 and 1920 as the interval during which modern medicine consolidated its professional authority.[7] Although struggles to establish appropriate criteria for medical training and licensing took place in state legislatures, courtrooms, and newspapers across the United States throughout this era, prior to the first decades of the twentieth century, acceptable medical education still occurred in a wide variety of for-profit institutions that adhered to disparate and often incompatible interpretations of medical knowledge. Some of these were relatively well-endowed schools, often affiliated with prestigious institutions of higher learning, while many were small, poorly equipped, and staffed by faculty who collected fees for their lectures. Yet, given the uneven state of medical knowledge in the nineteenth century, all were more or less heterodox in their approaches.

Beginning in the late 1870s, however, individual states began to pass legislation that required physicians to obtain degrees from legally chartered medical schools. Subsequently, the training requirements increased: first demanding premedical education; then extending the length of medical study; and finally, imposing postgraduate certifying examinations.[8] At the same time, a number of medical schools affiliated with major urban universities—including Johns Hopkins, Harvard, and the University of Pennsylvania—began to introduce new curricula that incorporated the laboratory-based sciences of physiology, histology, pathological anatomy, chemistry, and bacteriology then being developed and taught in Germany and France. They also extended the length of medical education to the now-standard four years to accommodate the new laboratory requirements. The transformations taking place in the laboratory and in medical education underwrote a new ethos in American medical practices that increasingly marginalized unorthodox or eclectic protocols, denigrating them as neither respectable nor legitimate—and hence no longer eligible for licensing—in favor of what came to be known as scientific medicine. In the process, not only were many medical schools that trained eclectics closed, but so were those that trained African Americans.[9] Hence, as Starr concludes, "The new system greatly increased the homogeneity and cohesiveness of the profession. The extended period of training helped to instill common values and beliefs among doctors, and the uniformity of the medical curriculum discouraged sectarian divisions."[10] Or, to put it in slightly different terms, the new system helped craft a new medical ethos and a new medical culture; it introduced a new mode of medical governance, both for physicians and for their patients.

The main manifesto for this still-reigning cultural ethic appeared in 1910 when the Carnegie Foundation for the Advancement of Teaching published its famous *Bulletin Number Four: Medical Education in the United States and Canada*, written by Abraham Flexner.[11] Now primarily known as the *Flexner Report*, the document articulated and elaborated the precepts that had begun to monopolize—and, many would argue, continue to monopolize—American medical education.[12] While often credited with establishing medical education on a scientific basis in North America, Flexner's report didn't initiate, but more accurately disseminated and popularized, the push within the profession toward standardization under the banner of scientific orthodoxy.[13] Yet, as I've already emphasized—and as its consent forms underscore—medicine is still not an exact science.

No doubt, the recent turn to evidence-based medicine has attempted to redress this inexactitude and to introduce greater certainty and efficacy into medical practice by assessing the statistical significance of health outcomes—albeit with mixed results. Nonetheless, medicine cannot establish robust relations between causes and effects that rise to the level of scientifically creditable correlations, let alone reveal the existence of reliable natural laws. Much as we might like to believe that medicine could someday achieve such certainty, perhaps by refining and standardizing its methods (i.e., making them more like algorithms) or basing them on genomic information (the promise of so-called personal medicine), it remains and will likely remain an improvisational and not a deterministic practice. In his mission statement for medical education, however, Flexner failed to discern any disagreement between medicine and science. Instead, he passionately promoted the notion that scientific medicine must supersede medical art as the basis for training new generations of physicians.

Yet Flexner himself was neither a physician nor a scientist (although his younger brother Simon, the first director of the Rockefeller Institute for Medical Research, was). Trained in classics, Flexner was an educator who had founded an experimental secondary school and in 1908 published *The American College*, which criticized the main methods of American higher education. This book highly impressed Henry Pritchett, then president of the Carnegie Foundation (whom Flexner congenially cites in *The American College*), who contracted Flexner to conduct the foundation's study of medical education in the United States and Canada. As Pritchett's introduction to Flexner's report makes clear, the foundation's interest in medical education was not modest:

> One of the problems of the future is *to educate the public itself* to appreciate the fact that very seldom, under existing conditions, does a patient receive the best aid which it is possible to give him in the present state of medicine, and that this is due mainly to the fact that a vast army of men [*sic*] is admitted to the practice of medicine who are *untrained in sciences fundamental to the profession* and quite without a sufficient experience with disease. *A right education of public opinion is one of the problems of future medical education.*[14]

In Pritchett's estimation—and it's important to remember that the Carnegie Foundation would henceforth bestow its lavish resources only according to the *Flexner Report*'s criteria[15]—enhancing medical education meant not just inculcating future doctors with the appropriate epistemological and practical tools to guide their therapeutic interventions. It also required training the medical consumer to seek out these practitioners because only they could provide "the best aid which it is possible to give."[16]

In the pursuit of this double-pronged pedagogical imperative, Flexner's report both offered proposals for the "proper basis of medical education" and propounded principles for promoting such propriety. Depicting the hierarchy of scientific knowledges that a prospective medical student must master, Flexner opined, "By the very nature of the case, admission to a *really modern medical school* must at least depend on a competent knowledge of chemistry, biology, and physics."[17] Flexner's prescription followed from the prior assumption that "the medical sciences proper—anatomy, physiology, pathology, and pharmacy" always entail the entanglements of these scientific competencies.[18] This premise in turn presupposed a layered set of expectations about vital functions that conceived them primarily as the biological manifestations of the natural laws that organic chemistry describes, which themselves incorporate the transformations of matter and energy to which physics attends: "The functional activities of the body propound questions in applied chemistry and applied physics. Nutrition and waste—what are these but chemical problems within the realm of biology? The mechanisms of circulation, of seeing, or hearing—what are these but physical problems under the same qualifications? The normal rhythm of physiological function must remain a riddle to students who cannot think and speak in biological, chemical, and physical language."[19] With this series of rhetorical questions ("what are these but ... ?") Flexner actually denies that these are real questions that might—or indeed must—remain open to interrogation, whether scientific or otherwise. Instead, he affirms biology, chemistry, and physics as the natural languages in which trained physicians must achieve fluency.

Needless to say, Flexner's characterization of medicine's proprietary knowledge base betrays the same understandings—or misunderstandings—of vital phenomena that Henri Bergson had tried to dislodge in *Creative Evolution* (discussed in chapter 1), published just three years earlier. Assuming that reductionism and determinism must guide modern medical education and practice, Flexner failed to consider that scientific knowledge production itself might not encompass all aspects of our aliveness. Instead, he embraced the experimental ethos that Claude Bernard began to propagate in the mid-nineteenth century as the justification for laboratory-based practices, largely founded on vivisection, to arrive at biological facts. Following Bernard into the lab, bacteriologists like Robert Koch and Louis Pasteur (who both trained as chemists, not biologists) then utilized new technologies (e.g., higher-resolution microscopes and staining media) in the 1870s to render microbes visible and intelligible as pathogenic agents.[20] For Koch and Pasteur, infectious diseases represented infestations by microbial parasites that they construed as the causes of these diseases.[21]

Imagining pathogenic microbes as voracious marauders that plundered an organism's natural resources, Koch and Pasteur held that infectious diseases represented the consequences of resource deprivation and depletion. Conversely, they assumed infected organisms were simply resource reservoirs—basically giant petri dishes of nutrients—on which pathogenic germs gorged themselves. Notice this narrative's key assumption, however: in this scenario, only the bacteria are active agents; the host organism remains entirely passive, appearing as a veritable *terra nullius*, ripe for colonization by invasive microbes determined to appropriate its vital reserves. By delineating these disease dynamics between active parasites and passive hosts, Koch and Pasteur invented the now-ubiquitous bio-logic that we familiarly shorthand as the "germ theory of disease."

In 1879, Louis Pasteur extended germ theory's bacterial bio-logic by performing a groundbreaking experiment in which bacteria that had been (accidentally) attenuated were found to induce resistance to cholera infections in chickens. The fortuitous event occurred when Pasteur inoculated a group of chickens with a bacterial culture that had been mistakenly left unattended for over a month (and thus exposed to ambient oxygen). He discovered that while the inoculated animals got slightly sick, they didn't contract the disease's more common and deadly version. The ever-frugal Pasteur, not wanting to waste his experimental animals, then had them reinoculated with a fresh bacterial culture that should have been fatal; yet none of the previously inoculated chickens got sick, while others that had not received the earlier doses but were inoculated with the same strain all died. Although he did not understand why this seemingly miraculous result occurred—at the time he theorized that the weakened microbes had consumed all the nutrients that the bacteria thrived upon, so when the more virulent strain was introduced, they had nothing to eat—Pasteur did recognize that the procedure had the potential to preempt other infectious diseases. As he later quipped about this discovery, "Fate favors the prepared mind." This fortuitous recognition provided the prototype for the first modern vaccine.[22] Capitalizing upon this fateful discovery, Pasteur proceeded to explore how to attenuate other bacteria in order to induce resistance to different kinds of contagion, inaugurating an ongoing quest for more and more vaccines.[23]

Despite this momentous technical advance, however, post-Pasteurian medicine's conceptual armory still unfortunately remained incomplete on its own terms. For even though the new vaccines were empirically effective, and thereby provided proof of concept for germ theory, the new prophylactic technology still left open a crucial question: if microbes are both pathogenic and ubiquitous, and if we haven't been vaccinated against all the possible disease-inducing microbes that surround us, then why aren't we all sick all the time? An answer to this vexing question presented itself a few years later in 1883, when a Russian zoologist, Élie Metchnikoff, writing against the grain of Pasteur's parasitic narrative, refuted the chemically minded bacteriologists' reductive renderings of host organisms as passive players in the disease process. A zoologist is someone who by definition appreciates the vital differences that organisms bring into existence, and as a zoologist Metchnikoff viewed the events of disease not as capitulations to predatory resource extraction, but rather as vital engagements among organisms of different scales.[24] Drawing on the bellicose metaphors that increasingly characterized epidemics after cholera, Metchnikoff reasoned that if an organism is invaded or attacked, it must necessarily defend itself. With this manifestly militaristic framing, Metchnikoff forged an unprecedented biological concept, "host defense," which he then christened using the legal and political idiom "immunity." In so doing, he made metaphorical sense of Bernard's all-out appeal for medical munitions for the first time.[25]

Metchnikoff's innovation proved crucial to the development of modern medicine by distinguishing it from what came before. As Georges Canguilhem noticed, in the wake of Metchnikoff's proposition that immunity represents an organism's means of maintaining itself against microbial predation, the *vis medicatrix naturae* lost its significance: "Ever since physiological science allowed the doctor to count on the existence of protective mechanisms of organic stability, it has become possible for doctors to cease invoking Nature as the providence of life."[26] Indeed, in his first attempt to elaborate immunity's role in the disease process, Metchnikoff explicitly claimed that immunity "represents the healing power of nature," thereby reducing healing's manifold potentials to just one: protection.[27] Over the last 125 years, immunity has become medicine's shibboleth. Any practice that doesn't favor this framework (e.g., acupuncture or Ayurveda) cannot be considered medically kosher. On the other hand, it is also why those of us who have been educated to esteem modern medicine now believe that our immune systems evolved to defend us against disease.[28] Thus, Metchnikoff offered a viable solution to the problem that germ theory created, and his defensive solution continues to underwrite contemporary medical theory and practice.[29]

Flexner wrote his 1910 report in the immediate wake of these momentous theoretical, technological, and biomedical developments, insisting that they provided the requisite groundwork for a really modern medical education: "Pathology and bacteriology are the sciences concerned with abnormalities of structure and function and their causation. Now the agents and forces which invade the body to its disadvantage play their game too, according to law. And to learn that law one goes once more to the same fundamental sciences upon which the anatomist and the physiologist have already freely drawn—*viz.*, biology, physics, and chemistry."[30] Flexner affirmed the principles of germ theory as the law that governs the game of life—whereas, in fact, only after Metchnikoff introduced the legal term *immunity* into biological discourse did germ theory achieve such a law-like status. Moreover, Flexner assumed that in order to understand the law that governed such pathological agents and forces, it was first necessary to turn to the fundamental sciences: physics, chemistry, and biology. In his estimation, these sciences provided resources for characterizing not only "abnormalities of structure and function" but also their "causation." In upholding this causal connection as critical to medical thinking, Flexner set out a program for medical education that has endured ever since—one that took (and takes) these sciences as a necessary and sufficient basis for explaining all manifestations of our existence as living organisms.

Unfortunately, in my case such explanations didn't quite suffice, since the manifold complications of autoimmune diseases in general—and Crohn's in particular—continue to baffle such bioscientific thinking (as chapter 2 underscores). My sense is that they might resist such reductive explanations not only because their causes have not been discovered in the laboratory but also because they might actually trouble the principles of fixed causality itself. We have known that questions of causality resist simple solutions at least since Aristotle, who introduced his fourfold plan of material, formal, efficient, and final causes almost twenty-five hundred years ago. Minimally, following Aristotle, it might have seemed that causes should always be regarded as plural. Be that as it may, we still often assume that an effect proceeds from a singular cause that precedes it.[31]

In logical terms, a definition of cause might go something like this: $x$ is a cause of $y$ if and only if $x$ precedes $y$ in time and if without $x$ no $y$ occurs. Or, to put it slightly differently: $x$ provides a necessary and sufficient condition for $y$. Needless to say, this form of monocausal or linear determinism (for each effect there is one determinable cause) does not exhaust the possibilities for describing relations between events that intimately inform one another. The causes of contagions highlight the conundrums that plague contemporary biomedical thinking, not just because they seem straightforward—a particular germ causes a particular disease—but also because historically they provided the model from which the belief that diseases have specific causes arose.[32] (Not to blow the plot, but . . . manifold uncertainties abound about whether such specific causes exist.)

The famous formula for fixing a specific microbial pathogen as causing a particular infection first appeared in 1890, when Robert Koch articulated the four criteria now known as Koch's postulates (or sometimes Koch-Henle postulates): (1) The microorganism must appear abundantly in all organisms suffering from the disease; (2) it must be isolated and cultivated in a pure medium; (3) when introduced into a healthy organism, it must cause the disease; and (4) it must be isolated again from the inoculated organism and cultured. Announcing protocols that could be used to isolate reliable pathogen-disease correlations, these standards also introduced and legitimated the notion that infectious diseases had specific causes that could be identified in the lab. The seemingly simple case of cholera illustrates the thinking behind Koch's postulates. Cholera was one of the first infectious diseases for which Koch isolated a bacterial cause (the so-called comma bacillus), in 1884.[33] Because the onset of cholera's symptoms could be both rapid and gruesome, the epidemics that afflicted Europe during the nineteenth century engendered enormous fear. Consequently, when Koch proclaimed that he had discovered its bacterial cause, he received prodigious public praise. This newly earned esteem, in turn, enabled Koch to push prevailing public health protocols away from initiatives focused on environmental interventions (e.g., sanitation, potable water, modern housing, uncontaminated food supplies) toward policies dedicated to controlling the spread of particular germs.[34]

Numerous revisions of Koch's postulates have been offered over the almost one hundred and thirty years since they were first introduced, as the many attempts to upgrade the principles of germ theory to changing bioscientific paradigms and technologies suggest.[35] Yet these concerted efforts to reconstitute causal criteria have not entirely clarified the connections between microbial pathogens and disease entities. Indeed, the picture seems to have gotten more murky, not less. For example, despite public health reforms and Koch's insights, cholera remains a scourge today, usually appearing where inadequate sanitation restricts reliable access to potable water (often due to economic, environmental, meteorological, geological, or military catastrophe). The World Health Organization estimates that there are between 1.4 and 4 million cases of cholera every year, precipitating up to 140,000 deaths.[36] Although epidemiologists still consider cholera a bacteria-borne disease, they are rethinking cholera's clear causal conditions and returning to the more expansive environmental explanations that preceded Koch. These include not only the political, economic, and social conditions that impact fresh water and wastewater infrastructures but also "global weather patterns, aquatic reservoirs, bacteriophages, zoo-plankton, the collective behavior of surface attached cells, an adaptive genome, and the deep sea, together with the bacterium and its host."[37] Given these manifest complexities, the supposedly determinate causal relation that has underwritten germ theory since Koch first crowned the comma bacillus as cholera's cause in 1880 can no longer claim complete coherence.

Given the inability of reductionist models to account for the convolutions in even this paradigmatic case of disease causality, we might need to reconsider our assumptions about disease causality more generally. If infectious diseases have so many precipitating catalysts and conditions, what does that imply for determining the causes of—let alone treatments for—chronic diseases? Perhaps the precepts that Flexner inscribed as the foundations of scientific medical education over a hundred years ago—and that continue to underwrite (in both the epistemological and financial senses) medical practice today—no longer suffice to answer this question. This is not to say that they might not continue to offer important resources or even that they might remain necessary. It's just that they might not be sufficient.

Even before I knew anything about Flexner's role in transforming medical training, this possibility first occurred to me in one of my sessions with Naomi. She remarked that in her experience as a student, a physician, and a patient, she often found biomedicine's reductive formulas unable to encompass the effects that diseases evoked either in her patients or in herself. This gave me pause, because until then I had believed that even though the cause of Crohn's was not yet known, it could in principle come to be known in the future. However, Naomi's comment made me wonder if thinking about disease causality in such terms can actually obscure the multiple determinants that coincide to form the events we think of as illnesses. Some of these factors must obviously include physical, chemical, and cellular precipitants since all life entangles such elements. Yet, because illnesses are not just diseases in the sense that medical pathologies describe but also life events, their determinants might also include a wider range of possibilities that cut across the lives into which they erupt. Thus, Naomi intimated that illnesses might have more causes than we currently imagine—if the concept of causality even fully captures the conditions of illness—and furthermore that how we imagine them might have significant implications for how we can learn to heal from them as well.

Visits to Naomi were entirely unlike any other doctor's appointments I'd had over the years since Crohn's first flared into my life—and not just because our meetings took place on a houseboat. Her ideas about what it means to be a doctor differed radically from those displayed—and espoused—in any of my previous encounters with physicians. The ways she practiced medicine changed my understanding of what medicine could be and made me wonder why more of it wasn't like this. To be fair, Naomi's method was far from traditional and not just medical. But that doesn't mean it wasn't also medical. After all, my insurance company had no problem affirming that it was medicine—they covered our sessions without any problem. However, given my previous unfamiliarity with this sort of therapeutic relationship, an obvious question arose in me: if this was medicine, what did *medicine* mean? And more importantly, what could it be?

To answer this question, recall that *medicine*'s etymology evokes judging, governing, and treating, so it always involves power relations between people. Hence, medicine doesn't only refer to the diagnostic and technological practices that physicians rely on; it also includes the dynamics between doctors and patients and the ways these are inflected by the former's knowledge and the latter's desires.[38] While some recent movements in medical education, including what is now called narrative medicine, have sought to elucidate the importance of these relational dynamics, by and large, medical encounters still assume that a physician's knowledge provides the most salient—if not an entirely sufficient— therapeutic resource.[39] But Naomi modeled a different doctor-patient relation that centered on helping me learn to heal rather than on trying to treat my symptoms.[40] Indeed, Naomi was the first physician I can recall who discussed the possibility of healing with me.

Among the resources that she explicitly brought to bear during our sessions, Naomi emphasized one in particular: psychosynthesis, a therapeutic mode she described as a "transpersonal psychology." Let me briefly introduce psychosynthesis, then, in order to sketch out how its effects on me changed the way I imagined the world and, even more importantly, my appreciation for how imagination shapes what we take—and perhaps mistake—as real. Very simply put, the ethic that underlies psychosynthesis holds that if you approach a doctor in the service of your healing, this indicates that the part of you that tends to heal is active and seeking encouragement and support. In service of your healing, the doctor's role in the therapeutic dynamic is to recognize and affirm this tendency. Indeed, unlike most modern medicine, which as we have seen has increasingly sidelined any interest in healing in favor of diagnosing and treating pathologies, psychosynthesis retains a strong commitment to healing as a primary process. Needless to say, although psychosynthesis was developed by a physician and can be practiced by physicians—like psychoanalysis before it—it is not, strictly speaking, a medical mode. Indeed, its practice bespeaks the recognition that as potent as medicine's knowledge often proves, it nevertheless does not always represent the "best aid which it is possible to give"—as Henry Pritchett promised in his introduction to the *Flexner Report*.

Addressed to the limits of this promise, psychosynthesis emerged from the clinical practice of the Italian physician and psychoanalyst Roberto Assagioli.[41] Born in Venice in 1888, Assagioli's life and training coincided with the scientific developments of bacteriology and immunology that Flexner posited as modern medicine's necessary and sufficient preconditions. Assagioli completed his medical training as both a psychiatrist and psychoanalyst in the first decade of the twentieth century at the famous Burghölzli Psychiatric Hospital in Zürich, Switzerland, under the direction of Eugen Bleuler (who, among other things, coined the psychological terms *schizophrenia*, *autism*, and *ambivalence*). At the same time, in Vienna, Freud was elaborating the precepts for psychoanalysis with his key texts *The Interpretation of Dreams* (1900) and *Three Essays on the Theory of Sexuality* (1905). The connection between Freud and Assagioli is not coincidental. For, although Assagioli never met Freud in person, he trained as a psychoanalyst, and the two communicated by mail. Moreover, Assagioli produced the first Italian translation of Freud's writing.[42] Yet, even though both were European Jewish doctors who entered into their medical practices during the bacteriological-immunological revolution (described above), they did not share the same estimations about its implications for healing.[43]

In fact, the notion of healing, which scientific medicine was busy retiring as its raison d'être in the wake of its biochemical turn, almost never appears in Freud's entire oeuvre. It was certainly not an outcome to which psychoanalysis ever overtly aspired.[44] The few times the word does show up in Freud's writings, it refers almost exclusively to an atavistic or anachronistic possibility associated with religious rather than scientific practices. In one telling instance, Freud clarifies his low estimation of the concept by establishing an equivalence among the motives found "in magic ritual, in tribal customs, in the observances of religious cults, and in the art of healing."[45] Magic, tribal, religious, and cultic are not terms for practices Freud holds in high esteem; neither, it seems, was "the art of healing." Moreover, since Freud took a famously secular and scientific perspective (e.g., he reduced his friend Romain Rolland's feeling of "oceanic oneness" to a form of infantile regression[46]), such associations doubly disqualified healing from Freud's therapeutic repertoire. Thus, while Freud once described the "lay analyst"—that is, the psychoanalyst who is not a physician—as a "secular pastoral worker," Freud's pastoral persuasion never diverged from his own secular, scientific training.[47]

Assagioli's pastoral work, on the other hand, did not adhere to the same strict limits. While his preparation as a physician also required imbibing the scientific spirit of bacteriology, immunology, and neurology, he nonetheless retained an interest in spiritualist or esoteric knowledges. Today such affiliations would probably seem to compromise any serious intellectual, let alone scientifically inclined, undertaking. However, in the first decades of the twentieth century, the immaterial or the unknowable remained viable concerns for otherwise enlightened thinkers, including the philosophers William James, Henri Bergson, and Gabriel Tarde, as well as the physician-psychoanalyst Carl Jung.[48] An avid reader of all these authors, Assagioli's interests in spiritual speculation did not succumb to his scientific training and remained with him throughout his life. Perhaps his spiritual affinity resisted his scientific training in part because he grew up in a household in which his devoutly Jewish mother also adhered to the tenets of Theosophy so that clashing precepts might not have been as troubling for him as they seemed to have been for Freud.[49] Moreover, Assagioli himself appreciated Theosophy, which along with Judaism he identified as his religious affiliation, as well as delved into several non-Western doctrines, including yoga and Vedanta-Upanishad philosophies. Given his investments in these more or less esoteric knowledges, which Freud insistently disavowed, Assagioli's initial affiliations with and affections for psychoanalysis shifted. As he wrote, "Psychosynthesis has evolved naturally, I would say spontaneously, from the ground, or out of the main stem of Psychoanalysis, as a method of psychotherapy."[50]

In order to appreciate this evolution, consider the way that Assagioli metaphorically invokes chemical processes, to both connect psychosynthesis to and distinguish it from psychoanalysis, even while underscoring his assumption that both techniques adhered to well-known scientific precepts:

> Psychosynthesis presupposes psychoanalysis or, rather, includes it as a first and necessary stage. There is in this respect a close analogy with chemical processes—both with those produced in the science laboratory and with those, even more wonderful, which are constantly going on in the human body. For instance, the complex molecules of the proteins contained in food are subdivided into the simpler molecules of peptones by the biochemical analytical processes of digestion. Through a process of synthesis, these are combined to form larger molecules constituting the specific proteins of our own organism. The same thing occurs in the human psyche, in which processes of dissolution and reconstruction are being carried on incessantly.[51]

Drawing upon his medical training, Assagioli's metaphor invokes the rules of chemical analysis (as defined by Antoine Lavoisier at the end of the eighteenth century, discussed below) which provided, and still provide, the investigative strategy that makes medicine seem scientific. Yet the chemical analogy also works to reveal the limitations of scientific medicine's analytic point of view. Noticing that organisms not only break down the complex compounds they consume but also recombine these constituents into new complex forms, he affirmed that the analytic and the synthetic, the "processes of dissolution and reconstruction," must continuously coexist. In affirming this resonance between the physiological and the psychological, Assagioli emphasized the need to recognize both the organism's constructive and reconstructive potentials. Hence, he indicates his belief that, far from being incompatible with the new biochemical protocols that dominated medical discourse, healing must remain central both to medicine's insights and to its aspirations.

Assagioli made this therapeutic ethos explicit in a lecture given in Rome in 1927 titled "A New Method of Healing: Psychosynthesis."[52] Unlike Freud, Assagioli had no difficulty associating healing not with anachronism, atavism, or magic, but with medicine's scientific state of the art. Moreover, he didn't succumb to the split of art and science that increasingly dominated medical thinking. Indeed, in Assagioli's practice, the faculties usually associated with art (i.e., creativity and the imagination) served as significant supplements to medicine's scientific ambitions. As he described the discoveries that he considered to have catalyzed the "radical transformation now going on in the field of medicine," he asserted, "The first one is the scientific recognition of *the enormous, practically unlimited influence of the mind* (in its widest sense) *upon the body*."[53] This recognition, Assagioli affirmed, offers a corrective to the biases that modern medicine had inclined toward since its biochemical turn. "During the period in which scientific materialism and positivism were the ruling influences, that is chiefly from about 1870 until lately [1927], great stress was placed on the influence of the body upon the mind, while the power of the mind upon the body was practically neglected."[54] Taking Freud's insights about unconscious processes to heart, Assagioli sought to reflect them back into the field of medical practice, suggesting that all illness—and indeed all health—involves the "'struggle for life' . . . going on among the various instincts, impulses, emotions, ideas, desires, and imaginations." This explained "why ordinary medicine fails in many cases and points to new and more promising methods of healing."[55] In the service of this promise, Assagioli advocated employing "active techniques" for therapy, including what has come to be known as guided imagery—or, as I thought of it when Naomi first introduced me to the practice, poetry therapy.

Guided imagery is one of the creative possibilities with which psychosynthesis sought to enhance the healing process. The use of directed visualization techniques did not originate with psychosynthesis, and Assagioli did not invent the many protocols currently in use by different therapists and practitioners. Freud himself had used similar techniques at the beginning of his practice (as he described in *Studies on Hysteria* [1895]), including the method of hypnotic suggestion developed by Hippolyte Bernheim. Moreover, a number of Freud's contemporaries, including Jung, also advocated active imaginative engagements both to circumvent the obstacles imposed by unconscious affects and to stimulate the "capacity to learn and create."[56] Inspired by these attempts to therapeutically engage the imagination, Assagioli refined their applications in the service of healing, developing psychosynthesis as a means to promote the power of the imagination in tandem with the power of science. Thus, never refusing the resources of biomedical knowledge, Assagioli instead affirmed that scientific rationality does not exhaust the entire realm of therapeutic possibilities we are capable of imagining.

The potential for images to radically reframe experience became palpable to me the first time I tried it under Naomi's direction. In one of our early sessions, as we sat looking out over the water, talking about some topic I no longer recall, I was suddenly beset by a series of sharp intestinal pains that caused me to catch my breath. Cramps were so common in my daily life that after I paused for a second to allow the waves of sensation to subside, I immediately continued with whatever I was saying—until Naomi pulled me up short by asking about what had just happened. I told her I was cramping, but I waved it off, saying it was nothing. You don't have to have read Freud's essay on negation to know that when someone says, "It's nothing," that usually means it's something, so being the good therapist that she was, she asked if I was still feeling the sensation.[57] I was, less intensely than before, although it was still quite visceral. However, it was not anything I couldn't tolerate, I assured her. And then she asked me if I was willing to try an experiment. (One of the key precepts of psychosynthesis is the activation of the will, so evoking a willingness to participate underlies all such interventions.[58]) "Of course," I replied, "that's why I'm here." She first asked me to sit back in my chair, to close my eyes, and to relax and then led me through a brief grounding practice—feeling where my body touched the chair as I breathed, feeling how my weight was distributed on the seat, feeling the floor under my feet, feeling the caress of my clothing against my skin, feeling the space around me, and so on—after which she asked if I could use my imagination to touch into the waves of contractions roiling through my gut. When I indicated that I had no problem making this connection, she asked me to conjure an image for the sensation. What occurred to me then, seemingly without thinking, is still as clear today as it was almost forty years ago: a wind-person.

I saw a small translucent creature whose nucleus was composed of pulsing forces in constant flux, spilling over and under each other but bound together by an invisible energy that held them in tension. This nucleus was shrouded in a veil that trailed behind it, concealing a wind-person trapped in a damp, narrow, cave-like tunnel from which it couldn't escape. The tunnel was so confining and humid that the wind-person feared its vital flames would be extinguished. To avoid imminent extinction, it rushed wildly forward, blindly searching for a way out. I said, "It feels caught. There's no room to breathe. All it can do is move, and the faster it moves, the more it has a sense of freedom. But when it moves that fast, it can't see the curves, and before it knows what's happening, it careens into the walls, crashing, tumbling, veering out of control, and that's what the cramp is, that crash." At this point, Naomi gently intervened (and I can hear the quiet cadence of her soft, calm voice as I write this): "But it's a wind-person. It can pass through walls. What happens if you allow it to expand through the walls of your intestines?" As she suggested this, I saw the veil dropping from around the nucleus, and the energies that had been bound together began to unknit themselves, to expand and diffuse across the lining of my intestinal tract, expanding through the tissues of my body, filling the room and then moving up out of it, out of the boat, floating gently up, up, up above Richardson Bay. Looking down from there, I could see the boat in the harbor, and in the boat Naomi and I sitting opposite one another in her office. She asked me what I was experiencing, and without hesitation I told her: lightness, spaciousness, breathing room, freedom. Then she asked me if I still felt the cramping, and to my great surprise I no longer did.

That set of images has guided me ever since. Allegorically, I have interpreted them over and over and over again in order to heal from many of the most difficult impasses in my life: physical, psychological, professional, political, and spiritual. They have revealed to me the ways I have frequently confined myself too narrowly, finding myself incapable of moving more freely, and risking injury and pain by trying to move too quickly instead. And they have reminded me that I do not need to accept these limitations, that I can allow myself to become bigger than I am currently perceiving myself in a situation, and that when I can see myself from a broader perspective, many more possibilities appear. Much like when the trances initially captured me while I was lying on my hospital bed—and perhaps also because of them—the first time I tried this active use of my imagination, it awakened a set of capacities in me that I never knew

I had. It helped me to consider that what I believed I knew about my pain, my illness, my body, when I considered myself as having Crohn's disease, was at best a very limited way of conceiving the situation.

Although Naomi was a doctor, she did not diagnose me. Instead, she asked me to discover my own meaning within whatever was occurring in the moment, not in order to know it as a specific disorder that might or might not be medically treatable, but as an experience in which I was participating. And perhaps this is what healing does: it changes the experiences that we have come to know as disease or illness, not only by attending to how these disrupt our physiological functions but also by altering the meanings we ascribe to them. Diagnosis—which, remember, means "by way of knowledge"—can provide important information about this experience; yet it does not tell us its truth. No matter what medical knowledge can reveal about the activities of our molecules, cells, and tissues, it cannot reveal what is actually happening to us because we are always more than these molecules, cells, and tissues, even if we are never *not* them as well. We are also how we imagine ourselves, whether we think so or not. The question is: Why don't we know this? And moreover, why in offering us its valuable insights and resources, does medicine encourage us not to know it as well? What happened to the healing potential of our imaginations in the modern medical imagination?

As advanced as it is, sometimes medicine seems a bit backward to me. For example, most of us probably heard about "gut wisdom," or "listening to your gut," or "gut instinct" long before medicine got around to recognizing the enteric nervous system—let alone the brain-gut-microbiome axis—as an essential aspect of our anatomy. And many of us knew that stress could cause hair to turn gray (if only by witnessing Barack Obama's radical hair transformation during his eight years in office) long before scientific studies confirmed this phenomenon. Similarly, long before the many peer-reviewed publications demonstrating that emotional states profoundly affect physiological function—and, not surprisingly, inflammatory bowel diseases in particular—it didn't require an advanced degree to realize this.[59] Indeed, it's not uncommon for people to recognize that affects affect their illnesses or that their emotions may constitute causal conditions. (Funny story: a few years after I was diagnosed with Crohn's, my father's best friend, Murray Cohen, was diagnosed with an ulcer. This was before ulcers were linked to a bacterium, *Helicobacter pylori*, as they now are, and were commonly attributed to suppressed emotions and stress—which despite the bacterial involvement may still be the case. Murray was a gentle, soft-spoken man, while my father was an insane rageaholic. After a family visit with the other Cohens, as we were climbing back into the car, the same blue Ford station wagon in which my bowels first unleashed their full fury, my father turned to me and said, "See, isn't it better that I express my anger and get it out, so I don't get an ulcer like Murray?" I silently screamed: *So, I have Crohn's instead?!*)

Given the escalating popular as well as bioscientific awareness that illnesses often entail phenomena that are simultaneously affective, imaginary, bodily, and biochemical, why doesn't orthodox medical culture incorporate this understanding more centrally?[60] Indeed, given that many of us have already learned this from experience, and that at least some bioscientists recognize its empirical validity, we might want to ask: Why doesn't mainstream medicine consider our imaginations to be more interesting, let alone realize that they might offer valuable therapeutic resources? Medicine's problem with the imagination—or the "imaginary problem" that plagues the medical imagination—derives in part from a conundrum that has plagued Western ways of knowing ever since Plato posited an essential distinction between appearance and reality as *the* problem that reason seeks to rectify.[61] Over the last four hundred years or so, let's say from Descartes onward, this classical philosophical opposition has been recast in a more modern mode as a disjunction between imagination and reality and/ or between imagination and reason. This happened especially in those discourses that aspired to profit from the soberness of scientific thought. Modern science engendered itself as such—that is, as both modern and scientific rather than traditional or dogmatic—by explicitly excluding the imagination from its field of investigation, which is to say from its domains of interest.[62]

According to this modern logic, the imagination can neither be verified nor falsified, so it can't reside "within the true" (as Canguilhem put it).[63] Instead, the imagination resists the true/false dichotomy that necessarily governs all (self-proclaimed) rational discourses. Hence, the imagination is prone to creating what Foucault called "teratolog[ies] of knowledge," monstrous ways of thinking that seem to threaten science from without.[64] Needless to say, whatever forms they take, such prowling monsters are by definition imaginary. To avoid the threats—whether imaginary or not—that such epistemic monstrosity represents, science continually tries to shore up the coherence of the true/ false distinction by purifying its knowledge practices of all potentially imaginary contaminants. As a result, the key epistemological questions become: What is the relation between the imagination and the real? Are they mutually exclusive?

Does the imagination prevent us from recognizing reality? Or might the imagination really exist? Moreover, might the imagination have real effects? Or, conversely, is reality only a figment of the imagination?[65]

More than two hundred years ago, the German philosopher Immanuel Kant pondered such concerns. Deeply troubled by them, he sought to reconcile the putative distinction between what gets called imagination and what gets called real in the second edition of his *Critique of Pure Reason* (1787). In response to the English philosopher David Hume's empirical arguments against rationalism, Kant invoked the imagination to bridge the conceptual chasm between sensation and understanding that Hume's thinking opened up. (Loosely described: empiricism holds that we can know the world only through sensory experience or direct observation; rationalism, on the other hand, believes that reason rather than experience paves the privileged path to the truth.[66]) Kant's *Critique* addresses the limits of empirical evidence to provide us with true knowledge about the world. It affirms that in order to grasp the world conceptually (as understanding) rather than merely apprehending it intuitively (as sensation), we need to organize and categorize the sensory data that we accept as given. Of course, here we might want to ask who or what gives these "givens"—for Kant the answer was clearly God—but that's a whole other ball of wax. However, as Kant observes, organization and categorization do not emerge spontaneously from the immediacy of the world. Instead, he argues that concepts, intrinsic to or created by human reason, can only correspond with sense data if the imagination links them by creating a schema that furnishes the forms and rules which govern this correspondence. Thus, according to Kant, the imagination, guided by its schema, limns the contours of our experience: "The schema is, in itself, always a product of the imagination. . . . This schematism of our understanding in regard to phenomena and their mere form, is an art, hidden in the depths of the human soul."[67]

Not by coincidence, three years before Kant insisted on the imagination's essential—albeit mysterious—role in human understanding, scientific and medical authorities were already busy trying to banish the imagination from their domains. The catalyst for this decisive move occurred in 1784, when the reigning French monarch, Louis XVI, appointed two royal commissions to investigate assertions made by the Austrian physician Franz Anton Mesmer that he could heal diseases by channeling a force he named "animal magnetism."[68] Today Mesmer is probably best remembered, if he is remembered at all, because his name gave rise to our word *mesmerize*. Despite our general ignorance of his importance (itself a result of the process that the royal investigations set in motion), the reports of the royal commissions repudiating Mesmer's methods

represent a watershed in the history of scientific medicine because they introduced an explicit distinction between real and imaginary treatments—the former constituting the province of physicians, the latter of charlatans and quacks.
Following Isabelle Stengers, we might say that the reports' debunking of animal
magnetism in the late eighteenth century served as the inaugural event, or the
primal scene, of modern medicine insofar as it claims to be a rational practice.
Furthermore, they did so at the very moment that the notion of the rational
itself was being tethered to the scientific.[69] Thus, one reason Abraham Flexner
could self-evidently assume that modern medical education must build on the
pyramid of physics, chemistry, and biology lies in the fact that 125 years earlier
the members of the royal commissions affirmed that physics and chemistry
constitute the necessary and sufficient criteria for establishing the validity of
medical practices. By assuming that the analytic logics and protocols of physical chemistry (which had just been invented) could adequately account for the
real effects that animal magnetism claimed to produce, the royal commissions
established a new scientific standard by which all medical therapies worthy of
the name still must abide.

When Mesmer first arrived in Paris in 1778 carrying letters of introduction
from the Austrian minister of foreign affairs, the understanding of who determined what made medicine legitimate or not, and by what standards, was in
flux.[70] For the preceding five hundred years, the medical profession in France
had been governed by the Faculté de Médecine de Paris, one of the *compagnies*
of the Université de Paris, whose traditional authority, like that of the university itself, leaned on the Catholic Church. The Faculté was a quasi-monopolistic
organization, financially and institutionally invested in its own centrality, and so
it often resisted new theories and practices, clinging instead to dogmatic frameworks derived from canonical Hippocratic/Galenic/Aristotelian texts. From the
Faculté's perspective, Mesmer's practice was clearly beyond the pale, given that it
involved a baroque apparatus called a *baquet*, placed in an opulent salon deco-
rated with carpets, mirrors, drapes, and tapestries; even more disconcerting, signs
of the zodiac were painted on the walls, and the salon was filled with haunting
music emanating from a glass harmonium. (I often consider this both a prototype
for the happenings and acid tests of the 1960s and a resurrection of the Asclepian
healing temples of antiquity—more about which follows in chapter 4.)

The *baquet* itself consisted of a wooden tub containing bottles of water
(supposedly) infused with animal magnetism, which were arranged in con-
centric circles, covered with iron filings and ground glass, and submerged in
water or damp sand. Mesmer then attached iron chains to the *baquet* to channel the magnetic flux, thereby allowing many clients to receive its benefits at

the same time. His mainly aristocratic and wealthy patients sat or lounged on upholstered benches around the *baquet*, wrapping themselves in these chains in order to direct the concentrated animal magnetism to the afflicted parts of their bodies. Mesmer himself, outfitted in lilac taffeta robes, attended to his patients by focusing the magnetic forces with his hands or with iron rods that he pointed at or applied directly to their suffering bodies. In these surroundings, his patients often experienced paroxysms or crises that, for many of them, ameliorated their illnesses and complaints. (For those who could not afford to participate in these séances, Mesmer also magnetized a tree near his residence, bound with iron chains that anyone could use to receive a free treatment.)

As outlandish as this procedure now seems, Mesmer actually modeled the *baquet* on the first electrical condenser, the Leyden jar, invented in 1745, which at the time was a state-of-the-art technology that enabled early electrical experiments. Indeed, Mesmer based his practice on contemporary studies of electromagnetism and derived his trademark technique from his earlier attempts to use actual magnets for healing ends. From these experiments, he claimed to have discovered a more diffuse, energetic animal magnetism that he could channel through various instruments, or through his own body, toward the suffering bodies of others. He held that animal magnetism exercised a material influence upon bodies through the mediation of a universal superfine fluid that sustains and embraces all animal life.[71] Illnesses, in his model, resulted from blockages of the magnetic fluid, and health was restored when the fluid ran free. Moreover, because there was a natural tendency toward this end anyway, the role of the mesmerist as physician was simply to assist and augment the natural tendency toward healing. Hence, in describing one of his early successes, Mesmer affirmed that his technique "had reestablished the ordinary course of nature and made those accidents which occasioned its suppression cease."[72] In Mesmer's view, animal magnetism, like Newtonian gravity, represented an insensible force that acted on physical bodies, according to predictable patterns—in this case magnetic polarization—to produce material results.[73]

Not surprisingly, the Faculté were not big fans of Mesmer's procedures—refusing to consider them seriously, especially after Mesmer openly ridiculed their motives and methods.[74] However, in 1778, the year of his arrival in Paris, a new rival institution, the Société Royale de Médecine, was endowed by Louis XVI with authority to oversee the nation's public health in particular and the practice of medicine more generally.[75] The Société's initial charge addressed the human and animal epidemics that threatened the nation (such as the rinderpest outbreak in the early 1770s, which decimated France's cattle herds). In addition to this epidemiological imperative, the Crown also tasked the Société with assessing the safety and effectiveness of new medical therapies (a duty that had heretofore fallen to the Faculté), which is why Mesmer's practice fell within their remit. To accomplish this second duty in a modern rather than a traditional way, the Société Royale de Médecine resolved to apply the latest criteria favored by the Académie Royale des Sciences (founded in 1666) to scientifically assess which therapeutic practices deserved its endorsement and which did not.[76]

Implicit in the Société's reframing was the assumption that its systematic, scientific methods and protocols offered a better means for evaluating potential therapeutics than the muddled, nonsystematic, backward-looking, traditional and theological criteria upon which the Faculté relied. Yet, while the Société simply purported to adjudicate the bona fides of new therapies according to these new standards, the effects of its decisions didn't just confer abstract epistemological legitimation on those it validated. They also, as Mesmer jealously but rightly noted, bestowed "encouragements, distinctions, recompenses, and prerogatives" upon them.[77] Thus, despite his obvious arrogance, belligerence, and defensiveness, Mesmer also had an important conceptual point to make about how the reigning scientific and medical establishments treated his assertions about animal magnetism. He insightfully asked: What "genre of proof" could determine the validity of his protocol? And whose authority would decide whether or not these proofs were sufficient to legitimate the treatment?[78]

At the time, the analytic techniques introduced by physical chemistry, especially as espoused by Lavoisier (who would become a member of the first royal commission appointed to investigate animal magnetism), provided the ultimate in scientific truth testing. The so-called chemical revolution of the last third of the eighteenth century—for which Lavoisier served as an inspiration if not a progenitor—invented new protocols for rigorous experimentation, which quickly came to provide a general truth standard for the sciences.[79] In Lavoisier's estimation, not only did scientific validity require experimentation, but valid experiments required him to exclude all variables not pertinent to his exploration, "*especially . . . the imagination which continually leads us beyond the truth [au dela du vrai]*."[80]

> The sole means of preventing such deviations consists in suppressing or at least simplifying our reasoning as much as possible, which by itself can lead us astray; to put it continually to the proof of experiment; to retain only the facts which are givens of nature and which cannot fool us; to seek the truth only in a natural series of experiments and observations, in the same way that mathematicians arrive at the solution of a problem

by the simple arrangement of givens and in reducing reasoning to such simple operations, to such succinct judgements, that they never lose sight of the evidence which serves them as a guide.[81]

In this mission statement for chemical analysis, Lavoisier indicates how the experimental method avoids succumbing to the seductions of the imagination, which "insofar as we are in some manner interested" would invite us "to seduce ourselves." Following the model of mathematics, he suggests, chemistry must proceed from one given (established fact) to another by logical linkages that are so limited they do not leave room for any imaginary insights or interests. Yet, whereas in mathematics givens are axioms that are supposed (or imagined) to be true a priori, in chemistry, or in any experimental science for that matter, the givens result from the reduction of a multiplicity of variables to singular facts. Despite this radical difference between mathematical and chemical givens—indeed, a bit further on in his text, Lavoisier admits that experimental data often "can only be known by effects which are for the most part fugitive and difficult to grasp"[82]—Lavoisier affirms an equivalence between them in order to assert the logical rigor of his chemical analysis. Thus, he establishes the criteria for making what will henceforth be considered scientifically interesting, if not true, statements.[83]

Mesmer actively disputed this methodology for testing his techniques and engaged in a public struggle with the Société about the principles upon which their evaluative practices relied. In a series of letters between Mesmer and Félix Vicq d'Azyr, the Société's perpetual secretary, published in the *Journal de Paris* in the summer of 1784, Mesmer made his disagreements with the Société's proposed testing protocols explicit by challenging the assumptions upon which they were based: "that is to say, that it is true that everything in the universe is isolated and that nothing is a cause and an effect at the same time . . . and that Nature and Medicine divide the empire of man in a distinct manner: that Nature can act on man in a state of health, but when he is sick, Medicine must act separately from Nature and outside the dependence on its first principles."[84] Then, not without a modicum of sarcasm, Mesmer concluded:

> Your Société, Monsieur, will surely develop its principles in a luminous manner; and a universe, built upon the system of your Architects, I have no doubt, will offer, in its brilliant incoherence, satisfying reasons for all the phenomena presented to your curiosity; because everything is connected, you will read everything with principles which isolate everything; you will construct your impoverished world, so singularly worked upon by our modern Archimedes, with instruments which seem first of

all appropriate only to destroying it; and we will be obliged to you for a new Physics, in which the ensemble of effects will result from the contradiction of causes, and in which the reality of some [effects] will give birth to the insufficiency of others [causes].[85]

Here Mesmer dissects the Société's interpretive method quite astutely. The Société, following the new chemistry, presumes that everything, while actually connected, can in principle—and must in practice—be isolated for the purposes of analysis. Moreover, he argues that this process of analysis by way of isolation presumes that destroying the analytic object, along with its networks of relations, provides the best means for determining the truth of material phenomena. Mesmer claims instead that his technique, predicated on interpersonal practices and intangible forces, cannot be verified—or falsified—using methods established to analyze chemical compounds. Moreover, he recognizes that the disqualification of effects as evidence of causes means that the criteria used by the Société Royale will necessarily exclude potentially viable and effective therapies, which might assuage human suffering, if it cannot identify their causes according to its chosen means of analysis.[86]

Because he objected to their methods, as well as their intentions, Mesmer refused to cooperate with Louis XVI's two royal commissions appointed in March 1784 to consider the validity of animal magnetism. Instead, the commissions worked with Charles Deslon, physician to the Comte d'Artois (Louis XVI's brother and the future king Charles X) as well as a doctor-regent of the Faculté de Médecine (until they expelled him for supporting the therapeutic use of animal magnetism). Deslon had been one of Mesmer's first converts in Paris, and for the purposes of their inquiry the commissions considered him Mesmer's proxy, despite the fact that Mesmer denounced Deslon for cooperating with them and also declared that in any case he had not shared all the secrets of his technique with Deslon. The first commission consisted of four members from the Faculté de Médecine, along with five members of the Académie Royale des Sciences, including Lavoisier, Benjamin Franklin, the astronomer Jean Sylvain Bailly, and the physician Joseph-Ignace Guillotin (of decapitation fame). A month later, a second commission composed of five members from the Société Royale de Médecine, including the botanist Antoine-Laurent de Jussieu, was also named. Clearly, the king and his advisors felt the issue of animal magnetism warranted considerable study by some of the most famous scientific figures of the era.[87]

The commissions in turn unleashed a flood of documents: each commission proffered its own official report;[88] the first commission also provided a "secret" document directed to the king (to reveal what they considered the more sala-cious aspects of animal magnetism);[89] in addition, they presented an *Exposé* of their experiments read by Bailly before the Académie des Sciences.[90] Besides its official report, the second commission also engendered a dissenting report from Jussieu, who, while agreeing with the finding that animal magnetism did not exist, felt that the commission's methods of examination foreclosed some therapeutic potential that the technique actually revealed.[91] Tens of thousands of copies of the main reports were disseminated by the Imprimerie Royale and the Imprimerie-Librarie de la Reine (some sources say twenty thousand; others, eighty thousand), which circulated widely throughout the country. Subsequently, these reports catalyzed a pamphlet war both supporting and opposing the use of animal magnetism, making Mesmer's therapeutic technique into one of the most popular topics for a periodical press already obsessed with the scientific advances of the era.[92] This wave of inquisitions, official reports, and popular representations, which led to and followed from the official debunking of mesmerism—and which finally precipitated Mesmer's quitting France for good in 1785—confirmed an ex-perimental protocol (isolate the unit of analysis), an experimental theory (only one cause per effect), and an experimental practice (blind testing) that continues to underwrite contemporary biomedical standards.

Of the official reports, the one produced by the first commission, reputedly written by Benjamin Franklin, had by far the greatest impact. The commission-ers, drawn from both the Faculté de Médecine and the Académie Royale des Sciences, saw their tasks as twofold: to determine if animal magnetism existed and, if so, to determine whether it had therapeutic effects. They quickly decided that if the first question was answered in the negative, then the second ques-tion was moot. To initiate their investigation, the commissioners had Deslon instruct them in Mesmer's theory and practice, which they then proceeded to try out on each other, but to no avail. After their failed attempt to emulate Mesmer's technique, they began visiting the *baquet* Deslon had installed in Paris, where they witnessed disturbing scenes of disordered bodies, which after a few hours of exposure to the magnetic apparatus began to enter into what Mesmer called "crises."[93] The commissioners were clearly amazed, although not convinced, by what they saw taking place around the *baquet*. The combinations of agitation and lethargy, the uncontrolled laughter and crying, and the precip-itous physical movements—shaking, rocking, wandering—seemed to testify to some powerful effects. But the commissioners decided that these phenomena could not serve as the basis for their evaluation because it would be impossible to isolate their causes: "too many things were seen all at once to be able to see anything in particular."[94]

The commissioners also quickly decided that they needed to exclude all collateral possibilities for the dramatic effects they witnessed around the *baquet* as well as the healings attributed to it. And the first thing they excluded was the healing power of nature itself. Since they admitted that "Nature cures [*guérit*] illnesses," they needed to assure themselves that the reported healings encouraged by animal magnetism would not have taken place without the treatment: "It would be absurd to choose in order to certify the existence of this agent, a means which, in attributing all of Nature's cures to it, would tend to prove that it has a useful and curative action, when it doesn't have any."[95] They then decided to follow Lavoisier's method of analysis in order to exclude variables, or "illusions," they considered especially extraneous by disaggregating the collective phenomena they witnessed near the *baquet* into a series of individual events they could more easily modulate and control. As a result of this experimental design decision, "the commissioners could only be struck by the difference of the public treatments around the *baquet* with the individual treatments."[96]

The first official participants recruited for the experimental treatments were working class (*personnes du peuple*), although subsequently the experiments were also extended to a "more distinguished class." Class difference turned out to be a significant variable, as only those of *la classe du peuple* felt any effects, while those of "a more elevated class, more enlightened [*doués de plus de lumières*], more capable of taking account of their sensations, felt nothing."[97] To explain this difference, the commissioners happily used their own imaginations to project what they imagined a working-class subject of their experiments might feel:

> Let us imagine [*Répresentons-nous*] the position of a *personne du peuple*, and consequently ignorant, attacked by a malady and desiring to be cured, led before a great assembly composed in part of doctors, where they [the doctors] administered an entirely unfamiliar treatment, and of which the *personne du peuple* was persuaded in advance that he [*sic*] would experience marvels [*prodiges*]. Let us add that compliance was compensated and that he believed that he would satisfy us more in saying that he experienced these effects, and we have the *natural causes* that explain these effects; or, we have at least legitimate reasons to doubt that the true cause is animal magnetism.[98]

Ironically, given their disdain for the imagination, the commissioners begin their analysis by imagining themselves in the place of the subjects of their experiments. They conjecture what these subjects might feel insofar as they would perceive themselves at the lower end of a simultaneously economic, educational, and professional hierarchy. The (needless to say) more enlightened members of the commission then assume that from their disadvantaged positions, the much less endowed experimental subjects, who also desired to be cured, would simultaneously desire to please those treating them. Synthesizing this series of suppositions, the commissioners then conclude that these supposed effects represent natural causes for the effects that (supposedly) accrue to animal magnetism. Or, as they affirm, "the commissioners are forced to suppose that these impressions, insofar as they were real, were the consequence of an anticipated persuasion, and can only be an effect of the imagination."[99]

Having made this imaginary supposition about the imagination, the commissioners then take it as a testable hypothesis that will now become the crux of their analysis: "It is necessary to destroy or confirm this supposition, to determine up to what point the imagination can influence our sensations and to notice if it can be the cause in whole or in part of the effects attributed to animal magnetism."[100] Just as Lavoisier had in his chemical experiments, they affirm the imagination as a cause, but only one that would contaminate the experimental situation. Hence, they determine that they need to develop an experimental design that can control for such unwanted variables in order to render reliable results. With their next subject, a working-class woman, they decide that since "it was only a matter of putting her imagination aside [*mettre à l'abri*], or at least invalidating it [*mettre en défaut*]," they will introduce a new protocol to do so: "Her eyes were blindfolded and she was magnetized."[101] Et voila, the commissioners invented a protocol that still constitutes the gold standard for validating new pharmaceuticals and therapies: blind testing.[102]

First, they magnetized the unnamed woman without the blindfold; then they blindfolded her and magnetized her again, but this time she didn't know where the (supposed) force was being directed. Finally, they told her she was being magnetized while she was blindfolded, although she wasn't. From her reactions, they deduced that "one can observe when the woman sees herself being magnetized, she situates her sensations precisely in the place that has been magnetized; instead, when she couldn't see, she placed the sensations randomly and in parts of her body far from the places where the Magnetism had been directed. *It is natural to conclude that the imagination determines these sensations whether they are true or false. . . . The sensations that she felt when she was not magnetized can only be the effect of the imagination.*"[103] The "natural conclusion" that the commissioners draw concerning the effects that their subject manifests while blindfolded indicates to them that the effects heretofore attributed to animal magnetism are in fact "naturally" effects of the subject's imagination. Although the commissioners remain resolutely uninterested in the imagination's nature, they have no problem assuming that it is natural and that it causes bodily effects.[104] The imagination acts, but its manner of action requires no explanation because, according to their methodology, it lies outside the domain of verification or falsification. Instead, they are content to affirm the imagination as an effective cause precisely because it allowed them to falsify the causal powers of animal magnetism.

The commissioners repeated their experiments on numerous subjects and elaborated new ways of blinding their subjects. In one case, they lured a working-class woman—known to have previously responded to being magnetized and thus to be "sensitive"—to a house under the pretext of a job interview. They then occupied an adjacent room into whose wooden door they had sawed a hole and replaced it with a paper facsimile through which they magnetized her without her knowing, thereby turning the house itself into a giant blindfold. In another case, they had Deslon magnetize a tree in an orchard outside Benjamin Franklin's residence while keeping their subject, an adolescent boy who was also known to be responsive to magnetism, under watch inside so that he didn't know which tree was magnetized. Reflecting on the combined data from their various "blind-tests," the commissioners conclude: "The experiments which have just been reported are uniform and are equally decisive; they authorize our conclusion that *the imagination is the true cause of the effects attributed to Magnetism.*"[105]

In elaborating the basis for their authority to assert that the imagination constitutes the "true cause" of the "effects attributed to [animal] Magnetism," the commissioners invoke a "rational physics" (*saine physique*) governed by the principle of sufficient reason as their conceptual benchmark.[106] In other words, they assume both that the logical standard that underwrites physics and chemistry provides a valid foundation for scientifically analyzing the responses of living human subjects and that this logic should therefore govern what we could call a "rational bio-logic" as well.[107] The commissioners thus presuppose that valid interpretations must comply with the principle of sufficient reason and, because according to this principle one cause is sufficient to explain an effect, if they accord causality to the imagination, they can therefore logically exclude the truth of animal magnetism: "Only one cause is necessary for an effect and since the imagination suffices, the [magnetic] fluid is unnecessary."[108]

Here the commissioners' logical dismissal is actually a double dismissal. For, in dismissing the effects attributed to animal magnetism as merely imaginary—even while acknowledging that the imagination can have real effects[109]—the commissioners simultaneously dismiss the imagination from the truth of medicine by conjuring it as the figure of the dismissible itself. To their way of thinking, the imagination must be excluded a priori from any scientific evaluation of therapeutics, just as Lavoisier had excluded it as a condition of possibility for chemical analysis, in order to arrive at the truth of material phenomena. Of course, the problem with transferring this supposition from physical chemistry to medicine is that chemical compounds don't seem to have a capacity to imagine, while humans do. Furthermore, sometimes when we imagine that we feel better, we actually do get better; sometimes our symptoms and suffering can be assuaged, even if not cured, as the commission's report even stipulated: "Without a doubt the imagination of the sick often has a large influence in the cure of their illnesses."[110] Thus, the imagination can sometimes support human healing, although it might not be able to assist chemical compounds in quite the same ways.

Alas, the royal commission seemed exceptionally indifferent to healing, or to the patients' desires to heal, let alone to be supported in their healing process. As a result, it disregarded the ways that the experimental subjects themselves made sense of their experiences.[111] While the way we make sense of our illnesses, or of the treatments that physicians can offer us, does not determine the effects that these therapies produce, it may inform how we participate in the process of healing itself. In seeking to elicit objective determinations about which treatments are worthy of medical approval, scientifically inclined medicine simultaneously brackets our subjective inputs by blinding us to our own involvement in these protocols. Indeed, the royal commission's blinding protocol served as medicine's first effort toward developing a scientific ethos—that is, to making medicine more like a science and less like an art—and its contemporary equivalents continue to underwrite these efforts today. While obvious advantages have accrued to this deterministic inclination, its epistemological bias may have unnecessarily encouraged medicine to turn a blind eye toward other therapeutic possibilities.

When medicine offers itself to us in its scientific guise, it tends (if not intends) to shape how we participate in the healing process according to its assumptions, often implying that the efficacy of its treatments occurs without much regard for our inputs. The presumption that medicine needed to promote deterministic therapies entered the medical imagination in the late eighteenth century along with the belief that the imagination had nothing significant to offer us therapeutically. However, bracketing the imagination is not the same as negating it. We can continue to imagine, no matter what medicine imagines about our imaginations, and sometimes what and how we imagine can make material differences to our experiences of illness. Nothing in any of my medical encounters prior to working with Naomi had suggested such a possibility, yet after my first guided imagery sessions with her, I quickly learned otherwise. This lesson has served me well ever since.

Although medicine no longer takes the imagination as a natural cause, that doesn't mean that it doesn't continue to recognize its manifestations, primarily by discounting them. Today, the notion of the placebo effect occupies the conceptual space against which a real effect can be tested, just as the imagination did for the royal commission. Not coincidentally, the first known use of *placebo* in a medical context occurred in 1785—a year after the royal commission published its report—in the second edition of Motherby's *New Medical Dictionary*, where it simply designated "a commonplace medicine or method."[112] Thereafter it was employed colloquially to disparage treatments understood as not derived from sound medical principles but rather dispensed in order to please patients and thereby curry both favor and income. (*Placebo* derives from the Latin verb *placeo*, meaning to please, give pleasure, be approved, be pleasing, be agreeable, be acceptable, suit, satisfy.[113]) Thus the placebo first served to designate the boundary of medicine by negatively characterizing the kinds of treatments offered by practitioners whom official medicine dismissed as "charlatans" or "quacks."[114] The assumptions underlying this usage are twofold: (1) there is a distinct though not always visible threshold that marks the difference between authentic and inauthentic treatments and, hence, between authentic and inauthentic practitioners; and (2) patients themselves will not be able to distinguish between authentic and inauthentic treatments or practitioners because they are susceptible to being "pleased." Needless to say, the same assumptions guided the royal commission in its endeavors. Leaving aside the implicit condescension and self-interest that percolate through these beliefs, one might want to ask, in what sense does a placebo "please"? For even if a placebo appears, biochemically speaking, useless (e.g., an inert substance or a mere nostrum), it still must have some efficacy in order to effect pleasure. In other words, it must appeal to someone or something in order to function as a placebo. Thus, we might need to inquire: To whom or what does the placebo's pleasure appeal? And how?

To speak of the placebo's pleasure is to underscore the elements of desire and imagination that it necessarily engages. After all, the placebo is not a thing, it's a relation.[115] No one gives themselves a placebo; a placebo is given. This reminds us that, in our species, experiences of illness often evoke not just cellular and biomolecular impulses toward physiological homeostasis but also an active desire for both relief and care. Moreover, they incorporate a capacity to imagine such possibilities—which is why placebos are not regularly part of animal experiments. If our reflexive capacities can influence the biochemical events that underlie disease and healing, then this suggests that our subjective experiences always already enter into the vital processes that we call our lives. In fact, from the current bioscientific point of view, our imaginary responses to the things that please us involve (at the very least) not only our neurons and the neuroelectric circuits that they weave, along with the complex biochemistry of neurotransmitters and neuroreceptors, including those in our guts, but also the dynamic interactions among all of these.[116]

Yet no matter how pleasing placebos may be or how they physiologically manage to please us, the placebo effect itself is an artifact produced by blind testing. In fact, it only emerged as an effect when researchers in medical and pharmaceutical laboratories started introducing ad hoc protocols to test new chemotherapies for streptococcal and pneumococcal infections in the 1930s, and subsequently for evaluating the first antibiotic, penicillin, in the early 1940s.[117] To verify the results of the new treatments, these researchers introduced nonactive controls into their studies so that they could comparatively assess their results against substances they assumed would produce no effects. Furthermore, they determined that if they made themselves unaware of whether the agents they tested were active or not, they could remove any taint of subjective desire for the protocol to succeed on the part of either themselves or the experimental subjects. Since the late 1950s, such double-blind methods have come to serve as the gold standard for evaluating new medical interventions. In these kinds of trials, the establishment of determinant causality for a specific treatment is based on the ability to statistically distinguish the effects of the treatment being tested from the effects of a placebo, given under similar circumstances, with the further proviso that those administering the trials do not themselves know which subjects are receiving placebos and which are not. Thus, while official medicine's current version of blind testing obviously doesn't rely on blindfolds anymore, it nevertheless still involves the same rational biologic of disqualification first framed by the royal commission in 1784.

While the idiom *placebo effect* reveals the imaginative and desiring aspects of medical treatments on one hand, it also tries to contain them on the other. In part, this tension between revelation and containment demonstrates a confusion between the two different senses of the term.[118] In biomedical discourse, a placebo is a control device used in clinical trials to provide both a standard of comparison and a means to ensure objective assessment. In this context, the placebo constitutes a procedural artifact introduced by a statistical mode of evaluation within which it affirms the possibility of determining, as a matter of objective evidence, the relation between the protocol being tested and the consequences that this protocol may or may not cause. Therefore, by testing a protocol against the results of a nontreatment control, clinical studies make the positive determination of a causal relation between treatment and cure into an actual placebo effect. The first effect of the placebo, then, is to affirm or negate the therapeutic potential of the tested protocol. Yet this procedural use of the placebo also gives rise to another effect: it demonstrates that seemingly nonreactive substances can also facilitate measurable physiological results. Indeed, double-blind testing is only meaningful because such results can be discerned, which appears to indicate that healing can and does take place independently of the specific protocols such trials seek to evaluate. The "placebo effect" here gestures toward a nondeterministic quantum of ameliorative agency that is recognized in the course of a study but that cannot be reduced to the effects of the protocol under consideration by "the rational relation of cause and effect as we conceive it"—as Léon Chertok and Isabelle Stengers put it.[119]

The placebo's inherent duplicity weaves through the history of its use. Ironically, even as double-blind testing produced increasingly reliable evidence of the efficacy of new treatment options—so much so that it has become essential to the approval process for new vaccines, pharmaceuticals, and medical devices, thereby engendering a global testing industry—it also provided increasing evidence for the consistently positive therapeutic effects induced by the control elements themselves. In 1955 a Harvard anesthesiologist, Henry K. Beecher, published a much-cited paper in the *Journal of the American Medical Association*, "The Powerful Placebo," in which he affirmed, "It is evident that placebos have a high degree of therapeutic effectiveness in treating subjective responses, decided improvement, interpreted under the unknowns technique as a real therapeutic effect, being produced in $35.2 \pm 2.2\%$ of the cases."[120] This widely disseminated, although probably overestimated, statistic seems to have underwritten a widespread acceptance of the ameliorative potential of nonspecific treatments. So much so, in fact, that it led not only to numerous attempts to explain the underlying physiological, cognitive, or psychological mechanisms that might account for such perplexing results (e.g., "conditioning," "expectation," "desire," "transference," "placebo-genic personalities," "opiate-mediated pain modulation") but also to a complete revision of medical history. From this placebo-centric perspective, it seems, any successes achieved by nonscientific forms of medical intervention in earlier periods or by nonmedical therapies of all sorts (including those that occur in other cultural contexts) must unwittingly manifest a placebo effect if they have not (yet) been verified according to current bioscientific paradigms. Clearly, this form of explanation serves to supplement a biomedical orthodoxy predicated exclusively on biochemical causalities insofar as it seeks to account for any nonspecific, nonreductionist amelioration of illness or suffering that has ever occurred by universalizing the "reason" that underwrites biomedicine's reign. Thus, it imagines that therapeutic treatments that took place before—or outside—biomedicine's hegemony can be explained (away) as effects of the placebo's undetermined or not-yet-determined causality.

Despite this prejudicial presumption, some physicians today still seek to exploit the placebo's unexplained and as-yet-unexplainable ameliorative capacity by expanding the placebo's role beyond the context of clinical trials to the treatment setting itself. The placebo effect, freed from the confines of the clinical trial, thus emerges to participate in the practice of medicine proper, albeit as a quasi-determined bioscientific protocol, and hence one potentially subject to objective evaluation. This practice, which relies on using so-called open-label placebos, has demonstrated efficacy in early trials involving inflammatory bowel disease, chronic low back pain, menstrual pain, postsurgical pain, depression, and insomnia, among others.[121] While explanations for why these therapeutic results occur remain highly contested, these studies are beginning to challenge the dominance of deterministic causality in explaining all therapeutic outcomes. Clearly, the use of open-label placebos in the clinical context remains marginal to most medical practice—although surveys of practicing physicians indicate that many doctors regularly prescribe placebos to patients without telling them. Nevertheless, the power of the placebo remains palpable in medicine precisely because it indicates—whether overtly or covertly—that medicine's dominant notions of causality do not necessarily encompass the entire range of possible effects that different therapies produce.

If we trace the history of modern medicine's rationality from the royal commission's debunking of Mesmer's practice to the placebo effect and beyond to the introduction of open-label placebos, we begin to see that for the last two hundred years the well-known ameliorative effects of the imagination have constituted what Foucault called a "subjugated knowledge" within the dominant medical imagination. Indeed, what this very long digression has tried to suggest is that while official medicine implicitly knows that the imagination can introduce demonstrable physiological transformations, it seems to care very little about them. No doubt, the length of my exposition reflects the fact that it's taken me a very long time to unknot the tangled beliefs about medicine that I assumed to be true before Naomi Remen introduced me to guided imagery. What Naomi offered me then were not only new ways to think about living with Crohn's disease but also new ways to understand what illness is—not to mention that she introduced me to the fact that healing can happen and that learning to imagine this possibility encourages it. Until my experience on Naomi's houseboat, my primary means of making sense of Crohn's had been given to me by doctors who adhered to the assumptions upon which American medical training and expertise have relied ever since the *Flexner Report* began to promote them. As a result, they not only had little appreciation for the imagination but seemed to have no awareness of—or interest in—its healing potential. Healing didn't figure in the ways they imagined medicine because it couldn't be captured by the reductionist methods which bioscience believes can entirely explain how human organisms live. In other words, my doctors didn't imagine that healing could appear within "the true" of medicine except as a figment of the imagination.[122]

Mainstream medicine continues to uncritically assume that its therapeutic powers depend on a conventionally scientific approach (i.e., one governed by the principle of sufficient reason) that brackets the imagination as a contaminating, or parasitic, phenomenon. Reading Foucault in the hospital had alerted me to the possibility that medicine didn't necessarily have to be what it has become and that other powerful possibilities for supporting healing might also exist. Indeed, as Foucault argued, one of the main problems with medicine's scientific aspirations stems from the ways in which it purges subjugated knowledges from the scientific domain of "the true" precisely in order to constitute its own knowledge as truth. Yet many monsters prowl beyond the professional and commercial boundaries that scientific medicine establishes, and in my experience many of these monstrous practices offer substantial benefits. Indeed, because some of these subjugated knowledges contain their own specific logics, languages, and demonstrable efficacies, they have been grudgingly reframed as alternative and complementary medicines.[123]

Acknowledging the unrealized potentials of these marginal and often uncultivated knowledges, however, might help us to discover other therapeutic possibilities that have been discarded or overwritten by medicine's faith in biochemical reductionism. Indeed, we might find that the seeming self-evidence of official medicine's scientific claims, while underwriting powerful therapeutics, nonetheless precludes other potent possibilities for encouraging us to heal and for supporting our healing processes.[124] Excluding the imagination from medical methods, then, not only might not have been necessary but may have diminished our capacity to imagine healing at all. Since its inception as a rational or scientific practice, modern medicine has implicitly recognized the therapeutic potential of the imagination, albeit only negatively, as that which it must exclude or denounce. When scientifically trained physicians like Roberto Assagioli or Naomi Remen seek to resist this exclusion—or, perhaps, to heal this wound—they come up against the limits of what medical culture has defined as the true source of its therapeutic power. However, as Assagioli noticed almost a hundred years ago, at the height of medicine's bacteriological-immunological triumph, a "new method of healing" might be possible. When he suggested that we appreciate "*the enormous, practically unlimited influence of the mind* (in its widest sense) *upon the body*," he encouraged us to reconsider that the imagination does not exceed the material, but rather that it always matters to us and in us—and so does healing.

## FOUR

# When We Learn to Heal, It Matters

It is a question of teaching and learning and not of disease and cure.
—MOSHE FELDENKRAIS, *Body and Mature Behavior* (2005)

Learning to imagine healing as both possible and desirable did not come naturally to me. Not only did it conflict with the Marxist-scientific worldview I had been raised on, but it ran athwart the historical circumstances in which I found myself living. In the summer of 1983, I moved with friends from the suburban sprawl that surrounded Stanford's pastoral campus to the grittier urban ground of the lower Haight in San Francisco. This was before the explosion of Silicon Valley caused the city's rents to skyrocket, so old Victorian flats, replete with cove ceilings, hardwood floors, and beautiful bay windows, remained within the budget of graduate students, at least if enough of us shared the rent. Of course, the location wasn't entirely ideal. We lived directly across from the overpass of Highway 101—through whose spans we could glimpse the spire of UC Berkeley's Campanile across the bay—opposite a truncated spur whose construction had been halted by mass protests during the 1960s. Beneath the highway, an unlit asphalt expanse served as an open-air drug and sex market; however, after the dealers and the prostitutes realized we weren't potential customers, they mostly left us alone. Just a ten-minute walk up Market Street from our flat was the Castro, which beckoned multitudes of queers from around the world as the Gay and Lesbian Mecca. In the year I moved there, it also became the US epicenter of the sexually transmitted condition that had only recently been named AIDS.[1]

The AIDS epidemic changed my life, as it did so many lives. When we first learned that a fatal, probably sexually transmitted disease stalked the city's streets, many of us felt the need to do something, although what we could do didn't always appear immediately obvious. As a young gay man who had recently survived his own death, I thought that I might have some experience that could be of use to others who were now dying. Through Naomi, who served as its medical advisor, I learned about the San Francisco Hospice and their work supporting those suffering with what was still being referred to as "the gay plague," so I volunteered. The men I met as a hospice volunteer had no illusions about what was going to happen to them. It happened so quickly that they could clearly see where their futures lay. By and large, the men I met as a volunteer "buddy" were deeply depressed, frightened, and withdrawn. Some were filled with fury, raging against the dying of their light. Some were already demented or catatonic. In those days their dying did not last long, and thus, as a hospice volunteer, I cycled through a number of men, most not much older than me. After a while, this morbid onslaught got to be too much death too fast, so I had to stop. It turned out that while I might have had some insight into being near death, my experience was nothing like that of the men I encountered as a hospice volunteer. After all, I had miraculously survived my dying, and none of them would. In such circumstances, the notion of healing just didn't seem to apply.

My experience also differed from that of the dying men I worked with in another important way, and that historical irony tormented me. Because I had lived with Crohn's since I was thirteen, including all its attendant bodily indignities and drug-induced side effects, I had not gamboled on the glorious sexual playground that inspired so many gay men to migrate to San Francisco. During my college years in the homophobic Jesuit enclave of Georgetown University, I loudly lamented my unwilled abstinence. When I moved to the Bay Area for grad school in 1980, I fantasized that I might finally find out what all the fuss was about. Alas, my health was so precarious during my first two years in California that sex remained off the menu. By the time I moved to San Francisco, after my third year in grad school, I was finally recovering enough physically to imagine that sex might not always remain such an impossible dream—but almost as soon as I conjured this dream, it vanished, as if it hadn't been a dream at all, but simply a mirage. Within the course of a year, the idea of sex transformed from a consuming desire into a terrifying if not deadly prospect, so I fell back on abstinence, my old friend. Even as I bewailed what I only somewhat jokingly called "my cruel fate," I did realize that it might also have saved my life.

I must have been going on about something like this in one of my sessions with Naomi. I don't remember exactly what I was saying, but it probably entailed railing against the injustice of my relentless sexual frustration and the unfairness of having such a shitty body. I might have expressed the belief that I'd been cursed at birth as well because the idea of having a malignant ruling spirit gave me some sense of satisfaction about my pathetic lot: if something evil was out to get me, not only was it not my fault, but it even made me special, albeit in a negative way. As she so often did, Naomi listened to my complaints with great compassion and then quietly said something like, "Well, how does your body feel now? Are you willing to find out?" Her quiet questions often had a way of shocking me into actually listening to what I'd just been saying, which in this case made me wonder what I'd meant, since obviously I didn't believe in fate or curses or spirits. When I assented, she began to lead me through another guided imagery session.

As always, it began with a grounding practice that invited me to carefully attend to being present and alive: appreciating sensations, sounds, breezes, gravity, breath, and pulse. Then, while encouraging me to hold onto that vital awareness, Naomi dropped in a simple prompt: "Can you find an image for what your body feels like right now?" The picture that instantly appeared was so apt it made me laugh out loud: I saw that my head had been severed from my torso but then clamped back on with an iron collar fastened by a huge, rusted padlock. Just as I'd suspected, I was a perfect Cartesian subject after all. Body/mind dualism, c'est moi, I thought. My mind just didn't want to feel connected to the rest of me. The collar that shackled my head to my neck both redressed and concealed a psychic wound that violently cleaved them in two. Furthermore, it so successfully disguised this separation that I hadn't even noticed its existence until that moment, let alone recognized the trauma that it represented. (Here's a flashback: as a teen, I identified with the talking head in a public service announcement paid for by the President's Council on Physical Fitness. In the ad, a silent, very buff man with a shaved head and dressed all in white carried around a box containing the head as it declaimed labyrinthine sentences clearly meant to convey extreme erudition. Lacking its own body, the head depended on the other's silent but very fit presence to move it from place to place. Unfortunately, by the time the head had finished pontificating, its bodily conveyance had exited the scene, leaving the boxed head stuck on the plinth where the brawny attendant had placed it, plaintively crying out for help. The tag line: "A body is a terrible thing to waste." Personally, I had great compassion for that head.[2])

Interrogating the image I'd just conjured, Naomi tried to guide me toward a stronger felt sense of mind-body connection, asking me to try to enter all its aspects and to incorporate their significance. But in the moment, my imagination would only take me so far. As I began to describe my discovery to Naomi, I realized that I wasn't quite correct in my initial body-mind interpretation. Descartes had certainly posited that the mind and the body manifest two different kinds of being, which he called the *res cogitans* and the *res extensa*, the thinking thing and the extended thing.[3] However, for Descartes the extended body was merely matter, a mechanism ordered according to God's plan, while my image had nothing mechanical about it. Everything below the neck was brutally alive, full of feeling and sensation; it just didn't belong to the head above it.[4] Rather, it seemed that the opposite might be true. Or, even worse, since neither my head nor my torso possessed the key to the rusted lock, perhaps we both belonged to someone else. Perhaps the collar didn't just hold me together; perhaps it also revealed that I was enslaved. (After a lot more therapy, I realized this was also an apt image for being held in thrall by the homophobia with which I'd grown up; I'm sure Naomi got that right away.) Although the image was incredibly vivid, I recoiled from receiving its full message. Repression doesn't capitulate quite so easily. Thus, at the end of that session, Naomi offered a helpful suggestion: perhaps I might be interested in trying out a somatic practice called Awareness through Movement (ATM), developed by an Israeli physicist and engineer, Moshe Feldenkrais, which encouraged neuromuscular learning by helping the mind become more interested in and attentive to its body.

At Naomi's recommendation, I contacted Chloe Scott, a dancer and a choreographer with a storied past. Daughter of a British naval officer, she'd participated in the rescue efforts during the British retreat from Dunkirk when she was fifteen, after which she'd been sent to New York to escape the London Blitz. There she studied with modern dance pioneers including Hanya Holm, Alwin Nikolais, and Martha Graham. In the late 1950s, Chloe landed on Perry Lane on the outskirts of Stanford's campus, just down the street from the wise Arcadian grove that set me on my healing path. During this period, Chloe studied with the experimental choreographer Anna Halprin and taught dance to children and adults, including 1960s luminaries Richard Alpert (Ram Dass), Stewart Brand, and Ken Kesey. In the early 1970s, Chloe participated in the first training that Feldenkrais gave in the United States and thereafter started practicing and teaching the Feldenkrais Method. By the time I met her, Chloe had moved around the corner from Perry Lane to Leland Avenue into what had been an old beer hall that had been relocated from a World War I training camp, on the back of which she'd added a dance studio with a wall of windows looking out over the shady backyard.

In Chloe's studio, I was introduced to Feldenkrais's learning technique, which, to my surprise—given my predilection toward dissociation from my body—comfortably conformed with my intellectualizing propensities. Because it encouraged me to use my mind to attend to how my body moved, it suggested that despite my long-standing mentalist proclivities, perhaps my body and mind weren't so distinct after all. Later, when I discovered more about his life, I realized this was not entirely a coincidence, since the method arose from Feldenkrais's active engagement of both mind and body in the service of his own healing. Feldenkrais had been educated as a scientist, receiving the first PhD from the Sorbonne as an *ingénieur-docteur*, a new degree designed to link developments in theoretical physics to practical technological innovation. While earning his degree he worked in the lab of Nobel Prize–winning physicists Frédéric and Irène Joliot-Curie. Just as significantly, he was also a judo master, selected by the founder of judo, Jigorō Kanō, to bring his teachings to European students. (*Higher Judo: Ground Work* [1952] was one of Feldenkrais's earliest publications.) Enlisting both his intellectual and martial arts training, Feldenkrais developed his movement practice out of his own desire to heal severe—and at the time inoperable—knee injuries he'd sustained while playing soccer.[5] In other words, his practice developed from his own desire to heal and to learn to heal, in the service of which he brought to bear both what he knew from his scientific training and also an awareness of what it hadn't taught him. Hence, for me, it turned out that Feldenkrais's method felicitously combined both the most overdeveloped and the most underdeveloped aspects of my personality, which was exactly what I needed to help my mind learn to think through my body in more holistic ways.

After a few sessions with Chloe, I quickly discerned that the Feldenkrais ATM classes had an overarching choreography. While there are now thousands of possible ways to organize an ATM class, Chloe usually began with us lying down, perpendicular to our habitual relation to gravity. Then she would suggest we make a movement, say sliding an arm along the ground from near the hip to shoulder height, which we would repeat many times. She'd ask us to move very slowly and to observe the range of motion and its quality, paying special attention to any places of sticking or discomfort, and noticing any sense of ease or grace. Then we'd switch to the other arm. Then we'd try them both at the same time. Focusing awareness on the motion and the sensations it involved gave my mind a safe means to become curious about how I moved as a body, and this curiosity allowed me a new entry into myself. (Feldenkrais claimed, "The only real quality that is innate in human beings is curiosity."[6]) For the rest of the class we'd introduce other movements that seemed to have little to do with the initial request to raise and lower our arms. For example, while lying down we might place our feet on the ground and rock our pelvises from side to side, then front and back, then in a circle in one direction, and then in the opposite direction, inscribing what Feldenkrais called a "pelvic clock." All the while, we'd be encouraged to observe the quality of the motion, to notice any limitations or impediments, to consider the differences between one side and the other, one direction or the other, and so on.

We used the least possible effort for these movements, inviting as much ease as possible. As a result, classes unfolded slowly, gradually progressing through a precise sequence of neuromuscular actions. Then, after these gestures, we'd return to our initial position and repeat the first movement, in this case sliding an arm along the ground. Invariably, at the end of class the movement was nothing like it had been at the beginning. The range was greater, the quality lighter, more fluent, more graceful, even though we had done nothing throughout the class to alter that movement per se. Instead, we'd implicitly learned that our habitual movements often include only a very limited engagement with our somatic potential, and, more importantly, that how we imagine what a movement entails might not encompass all it could be.[7] For me, the end of an ATM class always involved a moment of palpable surprise. I never tired of discovering that I was physically more capable than I'd known just an hour before and that by becoming more mindful of my movements, by focusing closely on their nuances, and by getting my intellect more interested in the body, which I'd thought of as distinct from my real self, I could cultivate that capacity more fully. Working with Chloe changed me from the inside out.

In addition to ATM classes, which lead people through movement sequences designed to disrupt disabling patterns by cuing new neuromuscular possibilities, Feldenkrais also developed another method, Functional Integration. This technique entails manipulation by a practitioner who actively initiates movements while the student remains passive, allowing the guided impulses to gently induce new neuromuscular experiences as well as qualities of motion. The practice of Functional Integration helps to revise deeply ingrained patterns of movement that we acquire as infants when we begin to rough in possibilities that we have not yet developed the muscular or neurological capacity to accomplish efficiently. Learning to walk provides an excellent example: when a child begins to walk, it has never walked before. It has never assumed a vertical relation to gravity on its own. It has never organized its muscles in order to align its skeleton to keep it upright in opposition to gravity, let alone to propel itself forward. Nor has it developed the synaptic connections that facilitate this peculiar bipedal muscular and skeletal orientation. Thus, when we learn to walk we don't do so in the most effective ways. It's likely that unless we retrain our neuromuscular capacities, say as dancers or athletes, the residual traces of the anxious, excited movement of early childhood will continue to characterize our adult stance. Relearning to walk with Chloe provided an amazing example of both what and how Feldenkrais taught: not only did I get taller and walk more gracefully—as my friends frequently exclaimed with astonishment—but I learned that even my most taken-for-granted ways of moving through the world had much more potential than I'd ever imagined.

Feldenkrais linked physical and imaginative development to their context, which he held was at once physical, familial, sexual, and socioeconomic.[8] Indeed, he believed that "a large part of the physiological freedom of the human nervous system is circumscribed by social tradition."[9] In discussing the way an infant learns to move, Feldenkrais noticed that a child's ambition to walk arises in the midst of adults walking around it. (Obviously, in different cultures, different protocols apply: for example, in some cultures a child will be carried for the first year so that it does not touch the ground, which alters its trajectory toward walking and institutes a particular culturally inflected, neuromuscular-psychosocial stance.[10]) Often the child's desire to learn a new activity such as walking resonates with the expectations of the adults upon whom it depends, and these adults might encourage the child to begin walking before it has developed enough neuromuscular capacity to do so without overcompensations.[11] These contradictory motivations can introduce functional limits that not only inhibit growth and development but also give rise to both physiological and psychological dysfunctions. That's why Feldenkrais argues that "maladjustment is not a disease, but the result of wrong learning or the learning of wrong methods."[12] Over time, these restricted and conflicted forms of use can become so habituated that we both take and mistake them for who we are.[13]

Feldenkrais proposed that we need as many sessions of Functional Integration as the number of years we have lived to undo the limited and limiting patterns we have acquired under conditions of dependence and anxiety. I was twenty-five at the time, so I worked with Chloe for the next year or so taking ATM classes every week and going for Functional Integration sessions every two weeks (again, thanks to my parents' bourgeois generosity, since needless to say none of this was covered even by my Cadillac health plan provided by Stanford University). After this intensive introduction, which radically revised the ways I both thought and moved, I considered training as a Feldenkrais teacher instead of completing my PhD, so I took a lot of classes and workshops with different instructors to get a better sense of the practice. Unfortunately, Feldenkrais died around this time (1984), and his organization fell into factional disputes, as too often happens when a charismatic teacher dies, so I decided to stick with the academic devil that I knew rather than launch myself into an unknown field rife with professional conflicts. Nonetheless, although I was supposed to be focused on writing my dissertation and jump-starting my academic career, I continued taking as many ATM classes and workshops as I could. I also began to engage with Feldenkrais's written works for the first time. Not surprisingly, exploring the concepts and insights that animated Feldenkrais's practice enhanced what I had intuitively gleaned from his students on a somatic level. More surprisingly, however, after I began reading Feldenkrais's texts, I soon realized how much Naomi's introduction to psychosynthesis and guided imagery had already prepared me to receive his ideas.

Like Assagioli, Feldenkrais moved beyond Freud by grasping that the imagination offers vital resources for both personal and collective transformation.[14] Indeed, recognizing that the imagination informs our human capacity to change—physically, psychically, and socially—inspired Feldenkrais to invent practical strategies to encourage and support what he called "the art of learning."[15] Both Feldenkrais and Assagioli recognized that our imaginative capacities enable us to innovate new neuromuscular and psychosocial pathways that can disrupt the sedimented routines we habitually employ to move through—and make sense of—the world. Moreover, they both proposed that by pursuing these new trajectories, we create contexts within which we can learn to live otherwise. As Feldenkrais succinctly affirmed: "you are certainly more creative in imagining alternatives than you know."[16] Juxtaposing creativity and imagination with knowing, Feldenkrais's practices seek to expand our repertoire of embodied and cognitive possibilities. Indeed, as I've been suggesting, inciting and encouraging this creativity offers a good way to understand not only what healing is but also what it can do.

And how do we become more than we know, if not by learning? According to Feldenkrais, humans do not just tend to learn, but tend to learn how to learn, which constitutes one of our distinctive features. Hence, he proposes, "The proper way to learn to do things is to learn how to learn first."[17] Obviously, many if not all animals learn in the sense that they adapt to and transform the environments in which they live. However, for humans, Feldenkrais suggests, learning constitutes one of our vital imperatives—it underwrites our earliest physiological and psychological growth. Following the intensive learning of early infancy, we begin to be able to imagine that we can become other than we are before we can actually do so. Thus, imagining new possibilities not only prefigures learning how to embody them but constitutes their condition of possibility. For humans, learning entails the capacity to imagine ourselves otherwise, and imagining means learning that we can realize other possibilities for living that aren't currently evident.

Because we depend on this learning dynamic both ontogenetically and phylogenetically, the imagination complicates what we take—or mistake—as real: "Is imagination a fact, a reality? Or is imagination only supposedly an imagined fact of existence? This may seem like just splitting hairs . . . ; however, it is a critical issue, as it concerns our knowing what we mean by knowing, what is reality, what is objective, and what is not. Above all, does it matter to me or to you, and if so in what way? . . . Movement, sensing, feeling, and thinking together make me, and the thing I am dealing with, as concrete and as real as I can experience."[18] Feldenkrais proposes the "fact" of the imagination as the basis for an epistemological and ontological practice that regards experience as the basis for human subjectivity. By imaginatively orienting ourselves toward the reality of the imagination—that is, by learning that reality and the imagination are not only *not* opposed, but entangled (as Kant proposed)—we affirm that we can always exceed what we currently take ourselves to be. Learning assumes a paramount position in Feldenkrais's thought because learning can also introduce a reflexive perspective, that is, learning can enhance the capacity to learn how to learn.[19] Hence, Feldenkrais argues that the potency of a practice depends upon its ability to foster learning, insofar as learning represents the capacity to surmount unnecessary functional deficiencies.[20]

As someone who had spent almost his entire life in school, I found Feldenkrais's insistence on the therapeutic value of learning a no-brainer. Yet, while reading his texts and studying with his students, I also recognized that my notion of learning had remained impoverished. Until then, I must have supposed that learning somehow magically took place in my head simply by reading a lot of books and writing a lot of papers. Learning just seemed to speak for itself—especially since it was something I got rewarded for doing without even knowing how I did it. Feldenkrais's emphasis on learning as a complex "cerebrosomatic" and psychosocial phenomenon challenged my unthinking assumptions: "Learning is not a purely mental occupation . . . just as the acquisition of skill is not a purely physical process. Essentially, it consists in recognizing in the total situation—environment, mind, and body—a relationship in the form of a sensation that in the long run becomes so distinct that we can almost describe it in sensible language."[21]

Feldenkrais describes learning as an entanglement of environment, mind, and body that we can sense. This dynamic conjunction belies the notion that mind, body, and environment can ever be experienced as separate realms. Much in our culture encourages us to believe bodies, minds, and environments remain distinct—including, or perhaps especially, our encounters with modern medicine.[22] Even our most intimate self-relations often betray the influence of these habitual misapprehensions of how we live. For example, in imagining my mind severed from my body and in identifying with my mind as the most crucial part of my self, I did not recognize that I had unreasonably restricted my notion of what mind means, let alone notice that I neglected the fact that mind is always and only an embodied attribute. However, when I read Feldenkrais's descriptions for the first time, I began to recognize that whatever I thought of as my mind did not encompass all that was obviously involved: "Mind, the unconscious, and the will are functions; they have no existence before action has taken place. They describe a relationship to a mode of action and nothing else."[23] Or, as he later underscores, "There is, therefore, no action that is purely mental, no thought without connection to reality."[24]

By insisting upon thinking and learning as embodied activities, Feldenkrais oriented his practice toward expanding the repertoire of human possibilities. If learning constitutes not merely a mental or social process, but a physiological, affective, and perhaps evolutionary one as well, then "the aim of education should be to help the individual achieve the state of an evolving being."[25] (This might be the aim of healing in its most expansive sense as well.) Thus, Feldenkrais characterized his pedagogical style as creating new contexts that could incite people to think differently in order to act differently: "The way I teach my students to work is to bring them into conditions where they can learn to think. They have to learn without words, with images, patterns, and connections. That sort of thinking always leads to a new way of action."[26] Indeed, he often suggested that he didn't teach at all, but rather created contexts that helped people integrate possibilities that would otherwise have remained unavailable if they remained fixed within their artificially constrained modes of existence: "I do not treat patients. I give lessons to help a person learn about himself or herself. Learning comes by the experience of the [physical] manipulation. I do not treat people, I do not cure people, I do not teach people. I tell them stories because I believe that learning is the most important thing for a human being."[27]

My engagement with Feldenkrais's work rearranged many of my synaptic and muscular connections, which in his terms is just another way of saying I learned a lot.[28] It refocused my thinking in both the general and academic senses. By introducing me to the art of learning and encouraging me to value my ability to learn how to learn, it inspired me to consider what learning to heal might involve. Although he titled one of his books *Body Awareness as Healing Therapy*, Feldenkrais did not often use the words *heal* or *healing* in his writings; nevertheless, his project suggested that both learning and healing unfold together. Moreover, it indicates that the latter always requires the former, that is, that healing describes a mode of learning. Or, to put this another way: it implies that healing always requires learning to heal. Whatever healing is, it is never the same thing twice because neither are we, so it seems appropriate that healing challenges us to realize that we are always more than we currently know or imagine.[29] Hence, in order to learn both to desire and to value healing, we might first need to unlearn the ways we have learned to imagine who or what we have been until now.

Like most Americans, until I'd come so close to death and then returned, I'd habitually imagined myself as an individual living among other individuals. In its conventional sense, an individual represents a being whose self-sameness seems self-evident. However, my experiences of acute illness and radical healing undid this self-isolating way of imagining myself. Since I could not claim responsibility for the things that had happened to me—I didn't intend to go into trances, or hear trees give me life-changing advice—I came to recognize that my so-called individuality did not encompass all that I am, and certainly not all that I could be. Feldenkrais's project helped me to understand that my individualizing tendency was not the result of ignorance or false consciousness, but was embedded and embodied in the limited ways I had learned to use myself.[30] Learning to heal was teaching me that while individualism might constitute the preferred political and psychological paradigm for imagining myself in the context in which I lived, it does not constitute a biological fact.[31] In undoing us and our most cherished expectations, illness sometimes provides us with an opportunity to learn to live beyond the limits that our culture represents as given. Learning that it is possible to live beyond these limits might indeed be one of healing's greatest gifts.

I don't want to make this sound as if this kind of learning is an individual responsibility. That would simply repeat the very presuppositions that modern medicine incorporates and that learning to heal might help us undo.[32] While modern individualism presupposes a primary self-relation that it imagines as a form of self-possession, Feldenkrais's practice helped me to recognize that the very attributes that I took as most intimately connected to my sense of self, the way I walked, the way I breathed, even the way I moved my bowels, did not originate from within me but came to me in the midst of others. In other words, I learned them so well that they became the basis for how I used myself as a self. Others always provide the context within which we individuate, and individuation always requires a relation between an individuating individual and the milieu within which it arises and comes forth. (I return to the complex processes of individuation and transindividuation below.) Indeed, the primacy of these relations to and with others serves as a condition of possibility for imagining ourselves as individuals in the first place. If we did not live in a culture which assumed that being an individual was the best—if not the only—way of being a person, then we would not be able to sustain this form of personhood. Paradoxically, one can only be an individual in a collective context where the individual serves as a privileged life form, that is, as a collective mode of living that singularizes and collectivizes at the same time.[33]

Feldenkrais's methods taught me that insofar as I imagined myself as an individual, my basic assumptions about being a living being remained impoverished, impeding my ability to realize capacities that exceeded both my individual imagination and my imagination that I was an individual. His pedagogical perspective taught me (at least) two things: (1) learning to learn and learning to heal constitute new ways of living, and (2) living always concerns processes that are not individual but transindividual. Together these insights inspired me to grow in new capacities that I'd never imagined possible before. Yet, as inspiring as Feldenkrais's teachings and teachers were, they still left me wondering how to incorporate their wisdom into my everyday life. How could I live these insights in ways that would enable me not just to continue to heal from all the short- and long-term side effects of Crohn's disease, but also to reimagine myself in the world so that my experience of Crohn's no longer constrained who I thought I was, or, more important, who I imagined I could be? And then, only after I managed to ask myself that question, and perhaps only because I was finally ready to receive them, I found new teachers who could help me to do just that.

I no longer remember how I got there, but after I moved to San Francisco, I found my way to a tai chi class taught by Savitri, a middle-aged Jewish woman who held classes in the basement of her suburban home, which she shared with her husband, a math professor at San Francisco State, and their very hip teenage daughter. Their smallish house, located in the fog belt at the top of Twin Peaks, radiated the latter-day hippie aesthetic still popular in the Bay Area in the mid-1980s, replete with crystal pendants and multicolored dream catchers hanging in the front windows and macramé plant holders overflowing with ferns suspended from the ceilings. Down a rickety wooden staircase, on an unfinished cement floor lit by a few bare bulbs, Savitri introduced me to tai chi's subtle dance. Her classes usually began with some basic qigong exercises to warm up and get the breath flowing before proceeding to a simple short-form practice, its pared-down choreography awakening bodily energies while simultaneously focusing our conscious attention. Then, once we were sufficiently invigorated in body and mind, Savitri would help us rough in a few new gestures from the long-form practice, which in its full expression could take fifteen minutes or so to unfold, taking it one step at a time (literally).

Although tai chi didn't captivate me enough to continue practicing for more than a few years, as a counterpoint to Feldenkrais it revealed another dimension to bodily energies about which I hadn't had a clue until then. Because Feldenkrais maintained a highly scientific perspective toward energy—not surprising, since he had trained in the laboratory of the Nobel Prize–winning physicists Frédéric and Irène Joliot-Curie, the discoverers of artificial radiation—he always retained a commitment to biophysical reductionism. Energy in Feldenkrais's perspective referred to the electrical, biomechanical, biochemical, and kinetic forces that animated and governed neuromuscular activity. Tai chi, on the other hand, arose in China from a non-Western lineage of physical explanation—c'hi or qi has no cognate concept in Western bioscience[34]—and it thus presented me with what, as an overeducated Westerner, I could apprehend only as a metaphor. Fortunately, working with Naomi had already taught me that metaphorical did not necessarily mean less real. Gradually, as I became more familiar with the practice, I started to sense tai chi's energetic dynamics awakening a new kind of kinesthetic awareness in me. Sometimes a diffuse sensory envelope seemed to extend beyond the boundaries of my skin, and in certain moments of intense concentration it even seemed to merge imperceptibly with those of the others in the class.[35] To my mind, the collective process amplified the energies in our shared space, creating a subtle field in which we all moved together. From that sense of an energetic field, I began to intuit that the boundaries of my skin might not constitute the boundaries of my self.

In anticipation of the Harmonic Convergence, Savitri organized a retreat at her property in Mendocino. Promoted by a peace movement, the Planet Art Network, the Harmonic Convergence (August 15–16, 1987) reputedly marked a fortuitous planetary conjunction that augured the moment when one cosmic cycle of the Aztec calendar ended and a new one began, ushering in a more peaceful era on Earth. While its supposed astrological significance seemed dubious to me (not to mention that it constituted an opportunistic appropriation of an indigenous cosmology), I wasn't averse to spending a weekend in the redwoods of Mendocino, so I loaded up my Ford Escort and drove north along the Pacific Coast Highway. Until I got to Black Oak Ranch, I had no idea that Savitri was an heiress. Her modest bungalow in San Francisco betrayed little hint of wealth. Yet she and her sister had inherited a lot of money in the 1960s, and together they bought a vast tract of prime Northern California real estate with it—a genius investment strategy, to say the least. They turned the old buildings and barn on the property into Camp Winnarainbow, a children's theater camp, run by the self-described hippie icon, flower geezer, poet Wavy Gravy.[36] They also built some new structures, including wooden geodesic domes anchored to redwoods reaching out over a creek running through the property, as well as a series of platforms, set high up in the forest canopy, between which they had stretched rope walkways that allowed one to travel high among the trees without ever touching the ground. Even if it turned out that the astrological conjunction had no tangible effects, between the trees and the tai chi, the workshop quickly transported me into a much more harmonic state. The resonance of the land's earthy and arboreal energies with those of the tai chi choreography, especially as performed with a large group of dedicated practitioners, amplified my sense of belonging to an energetic field that both included and exceeded me. Whether it was astrologically ordained or not, this convergence propelled me far beyond any sense of self I'd previously known and hopefully toward a more peaceful one as well.

The apex of the Harmonic Convergence was scheduled to occur a few hours after the workshop's end, while I was driving home. Just in case it might live up to the hype, as the most auspicious moment approached, I pulled my car over to the shoulder on a narrow road winding through a pine-covered mountain pass to honor whatever peaceful intention the moment might augur. I figured it couldn't hurt. In the heat of that late August afternoon, just steps from the asphalt strip where I'd parked, a small brook babbled its welcoming refrain. I took off my shoes and waded into the water, raising my arms to the trees surrounding me, thanking them for the blessings of their existence. Immersed in their *viriditas*, the vital wisdom of greening plants spoke to me once again and, as was their wont, the teaching was simple and direct: keep following this healing stream. At the time, I wasn't sure I knew what that might entail, but I felt its rightness coursing through me. Eventually I figured out that it probably meant that I'd need to keep going with that flow until it emptied into the sea.

During this period, my attempts to follow the healing current led me to consider dropping out of grad school on a regular basis. As far as I could tell, academic life did not seem to flow in a particularly healing direction. Casting about for a plan B, I tried out a number of options. Feldenkrais training was only one possibility that I tried but rejected. For one election cycle, I worked as a field organizer for the campaign to defeat a California proposition that would have limited social service benefits, including those for health care. In the year of Ronald Reagan's reelection, our victory—which merely meant that draconian cuts to benefits did not immediately take place—was a lonely bright spot.[37] Yet, despite the campaign's success, my despair about the larger political context made me realize that I was not cut out for electoral politics. I also spent considerable time exploring psychotherapy, completing a two-year psychosynthesis certificate program, undertaking an internship at the Pacific Center, a public mental health clinic in Berkeley for "sexual minorities" (as we were known at the time), and participating in several psychosynthesis work-shops led by Roberto Assagioli's protégé Piero Ferrucci.[38] I even enrolled in a clinical training program in holistic therapy at Antioch College, which in the end turned out to be a bit too touchy-feely for my excessively critical mind. I eventually dropped out of the training after others in my cohort kept inform-ing me that I was far too intellectual and not emotional enough, while I on the other hand kept insisting that emotions and intellect needed to work together to create more passionate forms of thought—no doubt we were both correct. Despite the failure of this last attempt to escape from academia, the experience nonetheless completely changed my life. It turned out that, although holistic therapy wasn't ultimately a good fit for my temperament, in the course's in-troductory module I encountered a charismatic teacher from whom I would continue to learn how to heal for the next thirty years.

On the first afternoon I met her, Emilie Conrad appeared in what I came to regard as her Egyptian priestess guise, her raven hair and deep-set kohl-rimmed eyes accentuated by an all-black ensemble adorned by a thicket of sil-ver necklaces—this exotic persona only slightly undone by a wicked comedic flair and the residual resonance of a Brooklyn accent.[39] Emilie came by her the-atricality honestly: as a young woman she'd trained with Katherine Dunham, the African American dancer, choreographer, writer, ethnographer, and activ-ist who established the foundations for modern Afro-Caribbean dance. (There are amazing photos of a young Emilie at the barre in Dunham's New York studio practicing next to James Dean.[40]) Emilie had then gone on to direct a dance troupe at a nightclub in Port-au-Prince, Haiti, for five years; traveled as a dancer with the filmmaker Maya Deren; and taught movement classes at the Ac-tors Studio in Los Angeles. In the late 1960s, she opened her own dance studio in LA, where she sowed the first seeds of a new movement practice, Continuum.

Emilie always said that Continuum grew out of her own desperate attempts to heal extreme psychic pain engendered by the cognitive dissonance between her long immersion in the spirited world of Afro-Haitian dance and her increasingly dissociated Southern California lifestyle. Intuiting that the clash between these antithetical modes of life would only be assuaged by expanding her repertoire of embodied possibilities, Emilie, dancer that she was, sought refuge in the organismic intelligence revealed by bodily movement. Continuum took many forms over the five decades that Emilie taught, some more formal, others more free-form, but they always preserved one initial impulse: life moves in and through us, and we must ride those movements, or we lose the wave.[41] Thus she taught that the more we recognize our own intrinsic movements and attend to their many manifestations, the more we can embrace vital possibilities for living that, because of our cultural and historical inscriptions, we might not (yet) have learned to value.

The first afternoon I met her, Emilie introduced me to what she called micromovements, which are the tiny nonvolitional and nonfunctional undulations of tissue that course through us all the time but mostly remain unappreciated because they do not contribute to the utilitarian modes of motion that Emilie sarcastically called "the hunt for food and the quest for fire." Sensations themselves mean little, she informed us; what matters (literally) is the value we accord to them. This was the lesson she'd learned from working with people with spinal cord injuries. Micromovements pulsed through their tissues all the time, but until they accorded significance to these slight perturbations and became curious about them—until they became interested and started to value them—these subtle movements made little difference to their experience. Yet once they began attending to these impulses, encouraging and perhaps amplifying them, people with (supposedly) irremediable spinal injuries often discovered potentials for movement that completely confounded their diagnosed paralyses. In Emilie's view, paralysis simply names a way of not valuing the body's intrinsic movements because if we're not moving at all, we're dead. In this sense, she suggested that we are all partially paralyzed by the values of the culture in which we live.

Emilie believed that in the United States, the dominant culture disregards movements that do not accrue profit in one way or another. This cultural bias, which defines the economic as our primary horizon of value, directs us to constrain our relations to ourselves and to each other according to functional, and increasingly mechanistic, patterns. (As, for example, when we work out on machines that repetitively guide our movements in order to give our bodies more definition.) When we incorporate these repetitive patterns of movement and attention, we restrict our ability to engage other apparently nonfunctional capabilities if they do not lead to outcomes that we deem economically, erotically, or aesthetically worthwhile. Conversely, since we don't develop bodily habits on our own (as Feldenkrais's example of a child learning to walk demonstrates), our habituated patterns are never natural, but instead represent embodied cultural values. To transform such culturally prescribed habits, Emilie taught, we need to create new cultural contexts that both affirm and support us in experimenting with different movement possibilities. By invoking and enhancing a field of significance that can support us as we explore such new potentials, these embodied value contexts help us appreciate capabilities that might otherwise remain unrealized. In other words, when we seek to transform ourselves, it helps to join with others to create collectives that can support us as we learn to body forth new ways of being.[42]

Emilie expounded a concept of mobility that vastly exceeded the strictly functional, one that sought to transform not only how we imagine but also how we experience our vital capacities as living beings. If we observe newborns before they develop much neuromuscular coordination, we witness cascades of micromovements. Infants' bodies undulate like waves rippling through water, the water that they mostly are, and since at one time we were all infants, we have all been immersed in this liquid state and retain its traces even now. (Conversely, one of the key aspects of aging is dehydration, so enhancing liquidity probably encourages vitality.) However, as we develop our neuromuscular capacities according to familial and cultural scripts—which, as Feldenkrais taught, diminish our range of movement potentials by channeling them toward particular gestures that we unconsciously repeat—most of us progressively lose interest in these early nonintentional possibilities, which seem increasingly unimportant. Continuum, on the other hand, holds that as living organisms we always retain residues of this original liquid potential. Hence, it holds that if we can learn to invoke and appreciate these traces, we can once again immerse ourselves in their fluid, creative matrix, perhaps learning to move—and therefore live—in more vibrant and graceful ways.[43]

Dipping into Continuum for the first time with Emilie woke up something that felt like an ancient, forgotten part of my mind-body.[44] Something moved in me of which I had no specific memory but which must have coursed through me as an infant and a young child, before my head got severed from my body image. Playing with micromovements invited me to enter into my own sensations, not as Feldenkrais had suggested (since his method focused on functional movement), but as a nonlocalized dance of intensities that radiated throughout my entire being. I felt a pleasurable quickening surge within me that sparked a diffuse joy which seemed to emanate beyond my skin. Having spent much of my adolescence and early adulthood in considerable pain trying to control the unwanted movements of my bowels that always threatened to undo me, it never occurred to me that uncontrolled bodily movement might bring such pleasure. Yet, as Emilie often reminded us, Continuum called upon the healing power of eros, not in the narrow sexual sense that our culture ascribes to it, but in the most expansive sense of vitality's palpable pleasure.[45] And after all, she'd say, isn't this exactly what babies teach us?

Despite the excitement my brief initial encounter with Continuum sparked that afternoon, I didn't immediately dive into it. It seemed like one of the many interesting healing practices that people in the Bay Area pursued, so I added it to my mental list of future pursuits. But soon thereafter, I learned that Emilie and her teaching partner Susan Harper regularly came up to San Francisco from LA, where the Continuum studio was located, to teach weekend workshops. My friend Rebecca (the one with ankylosing spondylitis, whose improper diagnosis led to two unnecessary and harmful spinal fusions) had also discovered Continuum and was so transformed by it that she insisted I check one out. That's how I ended up lying on the floor of a conference center on the Lone Mountain Campus of the University of San Francisco one Saturday morning, breathing, sounding, and undulating like a sea anemone.

While on her own Emilie was a stunning teacher, together Emilie and Susan took the learning to another level. Physically and characterologically, they were like yin and yang, dark and light, night and day, and when people said this (which they often did), Susan, contradicting her light appearance, always replied darkly, "Yes, and I'm the night." Susan had arrived in Emilie's studio for a weekend workshop as a twenty-one-year-old from Arizona, and in some sense she never left.[46] A petite, vivacious young woman with light curly hair and a pixie smile, Susan seemed Emilie's polar opposite, both bodily and temperamentally: shy where Emilie was bold, soft-spoken where Emilie was brash, restrained where Emilie was hyperbolic. Susan had been born in Rhodesia (Zimbabwe) to evangelical missionaries from southern Illinois who thought they were bringing salvation to the Shona people, but in the end the conversion worked in the opposite direction. Meeting Emilie, with her legacy of Afro-Haitian dance, reconnected Susan to her early years in Africa and, beneath that, to another way of moving and living that her American life had never supported. The week after their initial encounter, Susan moved to LA, first as Emilie's student and then as her teaching partner for more than three decades. An inveterate explorer of physical and psychic spaces, Susan traveled the world studying and teaching, bringing elements of Gestalt psychology, aikido, Rolfing,

Tibetan Buddhism, and African American healing and dance practices into Continuum. Her gift both for creating communal ritual and for tracking individual process enabled Susan to catalyze deep emotional and psychological transformations.

My first weekend workshop with Emilie and Susan converted me to their collaborative project. On the surface, what they taught seemed incredibly simple, like a return to what we all did in our play as young children. Combining intentional breathing, subtle sounds, and movement cues, they created a laboratory of sorts in which, by attending to the effects of these simple perturbations, we could begin to sense into the untapped and underappreciated capacities of both subtle and dynamic movement. Yet while these prompts were invaluable in initiating that inquiry, what proved most palpable to me in the process was the ambiance produced by a room full of people committed to exploring such possibilities on their own together. As we entered into this exploratory state, the collective space provided a supportive container that amplified our personal energies as we resonated both with each other and within ourselves. We used to joke that if someone passed outside the window and looked in while we were diving into the realm of sensation, they'd see a bunch of adults undulating on the floor, making weird noises, in absurd postures, and assume we'd all gone mad. Perhaps in terms of our culture's definitions of sanity, they would be right. For those of us who took to the practice, however, these sessions opened new vistas onto how to be humans living among other humans or, more simply, what it means to be alive.

Emilie was always quite clear about the political implications of Continuum. Attending to the subtle movements of energy that we are; taking the time to allow them to amplify in us; remaining curious about the differences they might make; and valuing the entire process—all these practices challenge the foundational assumptions of what Herbert Marcuse called capitalism's "performance principle."[47] There's no profit in practicing Continuum, no financial interest to accrue. There are no outcomes to measure, no goals to be met, and time is definitely not money. You will not end up sexier, richer, or fitter, or at least not intentionally. (And, of course, it costs money to enroll—so in capitalism's terms, it's definitely a bad investment.) Instead, Continuum calls on us to question the ontological and epistemological premises underlying the appropriative political and economic systems that dominate our culture and increasingly our world—even if we still have to pay to learn this lesson (since we still live within capitalism, after all).

Here's an example: one of Emilie's favorite sayings was "in movement there are no objects," an insight that subverts the subject/object dichotomy that underwrites the scientific and technological paradigms on which our economic systems increasingly depend. In other words, if we do not objectify ourselves or allow ourselves to be objectified, and if we realize that movement is not what we do but what we are, then it becomes harder to buy into the premises that underwrite capitalism's reigning ideology of possessive individualism (i.e., that we have bodies that we possess as property and whose labor power we can contractually lease to employers in exchange for wages).[48] Moreover, it teaches us that we are not fundamentally disconnected from others or from the planet and only belatedly related to each other through social contracts or economic relations. It refuses to accept the notion that we can exist without coexisting or that the enhancement of one's life comes only at the expense of others. Rather, it viscerally demonstrates that as living beings we are all transformations of matter and energy localized in time and space and that, for the duration we call a lifetime, we are always on the move together—whether we like it or not.

We lose our connections with our early vitality only because we learn that we must channel our energies into more productive patterns in order to become viable economic and psychosexual subjects. For, as Feldenkrais reminded us, "The problem is that much of what we learned is harmful to our system, because it was learned in childhood, when immediate dependence on others distorted our real needs."[49] Therefore, when we attend schools that teach us that we must sit down, shut up, and pay attention to a teacher in order to acquire the cognitive skills that will allow us to emerge as employable adults, we also learn that our movement capacities must be disciplined in order to be worthwhile—as children diagnosed with ADHD or autism know too well.[50] Maintaining such restrictive bodily habits and mindsets requires us not only to willfully not know and not feel but also to willfully not value some of the most vital attributes we were born with. Luckily for us, no matter how suppressed they might become, these animated impulses persist—because, as Bergson reminds us, "the essence of life is in the movement by which life is transmitted." Thus, given sufficient resources, support, and encouragement, we retain the capacity to recall it, if and when we so desire.

Although I immediately apprehended the significance of Continuum on a gut level, I didn't necessarily understand why. The conceptual paradigms I'd been learning about in my scholarly training certainly didn't provide an adequate frame for my experience—which is not surprising since Continuum actively challenged most of them. Only when I discovered the work of the French philosopher

Gilbert Simondon after almost two decades of practicing Continuum did I finally discover intellectual tools that could help me elucidate its lessons. Although he himself might not have recognized the connection, Simondon's writings helped me explain why Continuum's convivial contexts could catalyze a transformational field by establishing what Simondon called an "internal resonance" within our collective practice.[51] Simondon's notion of internal resonance offered me a way to think about the healing potentials that Continuum both evoked and expressed. After all, in workshops we intentionally created contexts in which we actually resonated with each other—using breath, voice, and gesture—and in so doing we called in unanticipated ways of moving and living together. These workshops encompassed fields of possibilities that too often remained elusive in daily life, given that our everyday lives were so bound up with imperatives of subsistence and survival in late capitalism. Because Continuum explicitly amplified and condensed the vital movements that always pulse within us, albeit usually without much recognition or appreciation, the internal resonance it created enabled me to start to resolve—and to heal—problems that plagued me as long as I regarded myself as an isolated individual who had Crohn's.

Simondon was a mid-twentieth-century French philosopher who studied with Georges Canguilhem as well as the phenomenologist Maurice Merleau-Ponty. In his 1958 doctoral dissertation, "L'individuation à la lumière des notions de forme et d'information," Simondon undertook a radical revision of the ontotheology that has underwritten Western thinking about living beings at least since Aristotle. (Ontotheology is the name Martin Heidegger gave to the habits of thought that emerged in Greek antiquity for apprehending "true knowledge" about the world and that have persisted in various guises since then.[52]) Some people prefer to call this way of thinking metaphysics. These modes of thought suggest that what matters most in the world, and in our lives, always exceeds how we perceive the matter that we are.[53] This perspective gives rise to an opposition between appearance and reality that Western philosophy has attempted to rectify for over two thousand years. From this philosophical point of view, discerning what remains nonapparent in what we (mis)take as real constitutes the proper activity of reason. To grasp such nonapparent aspects of reality, we must develop concepts (from the Latin: con + capere, to take hold of or seize with), and in Western thought these concepts frequently appear as conjoint opposites: true/false, good/bad, male/female, right/wrong, and so on.[54]

Perhaps the best-known—and the most consequential—of these conceptual oppositions is body/soul, first introduced by Plato in the *Phaedo*, his dialogue on the death of Socrates.[55] Plato's erstwhile student, Aristotle, then reframed Plato's body/soul opposition and offered a different but related conceptual pairing that also remains deeply embedded in Western modes of thinking: form/matter. Called hylomorphism, this Aristotelian doctrine conceives of any individual being as a compound of matter and form.[56] The most famous example used to explain hylomorphism is a brick: from the hylomorphic perspective, a brick is a brick because matter (mud) is placed in a form (a mold) in which it hardens into a brick. According to this schema, the mud is its potentiality, the mold its actuality. In the case of humans, hylomorphism holds that our matter (the body) is imbued with a form (the soul), and their compound determines us as the living beings we are.[57]

Simondon's revision of Western ontotheology begins by troubling hylomorphism's binary terms as a means for thinking about individuated beings. Rather than take beings as composed of form and matter, or soul and body, Simondon recognized that such bifurcating schemata leave out something essential. Consider the brick: a brick is not just mud slapped into a mold. Rather, the energy from the kiln enables the mud in the rectilinear mold to assume and retain the form of the brick.[58] When you tell a story about how to build a house in terms of individual bricks, you forget the energy, as well as the labor, as well as the place the mud comes from, as well as the insight that inspired the technology, as well as the other animals and plants displaced by the kiln and the aggregations of humans needed to run the kiln, as well as the trees, or the coal, needed to fire the kiln—but you get my drift.

Rather than focus on the brick, or the person, as an individual, Simondon suggests that we need to rethink individuals as constituting phases in processes of individuation. These phases arise out of what he names the "preindividual" (in which "form, matter, and energy preexist in the system"), and they will eventually fall out of phase with themselves (*se dephaser*).[59] According to Simondon, individuals—whether crystals, bricks, humans, nations, planets, or galaxies— emerge as temporary resolutions of tensions that exist in a preindividual plenitude of potentials, including some potentials which are mutually exclusive, such that no individual can ever realize all these preindividual possibilities. In other words, the individuated person proceeds from something that both precedes and exceeds it. Moreover, it carries within it traces of that preindividual abundance that came before and which continues to unfold within it. Some of these traces include preindividual "forces in tension" that give rise to "problems" which a living being then might seek to resolve.

As Simondon puts it: the preindividual is "more than a unity," and he recruits a term from modern physics, "metastability," to characterize this "more than."[60] (Metastability refers to the relative stability of a far-from-equilibrium system. In such a dynamic system, the potential energy in the system has not been exhausted, and so it retains the capacity for further transformations.) In this sense, the metastable preindividual constitutes "the initial supersaturation of being" before individuation, and as such it is both not-one and more-than-one.[61] Think here of the big bang, or the first cell springing into being from an oceanic soup, or of the totipotency of a fertilized egg. The state from which a system arises, whether we're talking about the universe, all life, or a single living being, contains many more possibilities than any individuated being itself can realize, and this excess persists by way of these (as yet) unrealized potentials. By conceiving of the preindividual as an abundance from which any and all individuated beings must arise, Simondon reframes how we think the individual per se: "Individuation must be thought then as a partial and relative resolution that occurs in a system which receives its potentials and contains a certain incompatibility in relation to itself, an incompatibility composed of forces in tension as well as the impossibility of interaction between terms of extreme dimensions."[62] Simondon's insight helps us recognize the limits of imagining beings—all beings, any beings, including human beings—first and foremost as individuals. What we think of as individuals are better understood as phases that crystallize within a play of forces whose consistency always includes possibilities that tend to undo or "fall out of phase with [*se dephaser*]" themselves.

When we fix these phases as entities, as individuals, we restrict our attention to instances of relative and partial stability within the system, forgetting that this stability is not an equilibrium but a metastability from which it will inevitably depart, as all far-from-equilibrium systems do.[63] If we don't assume the self-evidence of the individual as such, however, we can begin to recognize the complicated dynamics always in play throughout the ongoing course of individuation. Focusing on individuation, instead of taking individuals as given, foregrounds the ongoingness of the processes through which our going-on-living takes place. The Continuum shorthand for this is: we are never fully born; we are always in the birthing process—until and even perhaps when we die. Or, to translate into Simondon's terms: we are not individuals, we are always individuating—until we fall out of phase with ourselves as living beings and die.

This lively insight helps us recognize that as individuals we are never autonomous: "The individual would then be grasped as a relative reality, a certain phase of the being that supposes a preindividual reality, and which even after individuation does not exist by itself, because individuation does not exhaust the potentials of the preindividual reality all at once, and because what individuation makes appear is not only the individual but the individual-milieu dyad."[64] Individuation always gives rise to more than just individuals, since individuals exist only in contexts, and those contexts are necessarily part of what an individual is. In the case of living beings, this entanglement propels an organism to transform itself by continuing to individuate itself but always in situ: "There is in the living an individuation by the individual. . . . The living resolves problems not only in adapting itself, that is by modifying its relations to the milieu (which a machine can do), but by modifying itself, by inventing new internal structures and introducing itself completely into vital problems. The living individual is a system of individuation, an individuating system, and a system which individuates itself."[65]

For humans, the individuating systems that we are and in which we participate are simultaneously physical, vital, psychic, and social. As living beings, we individuate at each of these scales simultaneously, and the tensions they set in play give rise to problems, the resolution of which impels our further individuation: "The living, which is at once both more and less than a unity, carries with it an inner problematic, and as an element can enter into a problematic much larger than its own being. Participation, for the individual, is the fact of being an element in a much larger individuation by the intermediary of the preindividual reality that the individual contains, that is to say, thanks to the potentials it receives."[66] How we participate as living beings who are also human entails both how we individuate (within) ourselves and how we individuate with others. Thus, following Simondon, it might be more accurate to think of ourselves as particulars and participants rather than individuals and agents, as the dominant worldview of contemporary capitalism encourages us to do. The dimensions of our individuation as living human beings who are both psychic and social remain entangled with all other beings, both animate and inanimate (as Spinoza underscored). When confronted with problems as living beings, we can resolve them only insofar as we address them on all levels simultaneously. As a consequence, for humans, vital individuation also entails psychic and social individuations that, through a dimension Simondon calls the "transindividual," give rise to individuals who are "group individuals."[67]

Kin, clans, tribes, sects, nations, religions, classes, corporations, organizations, and political movements all provide examples of transindividuation insofar as they establish and maintain internal resonances that reverberate throughout a group and thereby engender and maintain its consistence.[68] By virtue of the psyche's mediation between the vital and the social, between the preindividual and the transindividual, it calls for—and sometimes calls forth—collective resolutions to its problems. Without such collective resonance and resolution, Simondon argues, individuals as such can never surmount our problems, and instead we fall back into anxiety because as humans we weave together multiple dimensions of being that remain in tension, if isolated at the level of the individual.[69]

Of course, this is also what both psychoanalysis and psychosynthesis under-stood. Our existence as living human beings evokes conflicts between organic impulses and cultural prescriptions, giving rise to the fraught psychic drama of the individual that Freud famously elucidated in *Civilization and Its Discontents*.[70] Furthermore, individuation for Freud is a traumatic process that requires the infant's more or less violent exit from the biological and psychic dependency of its early life as well as the repression of those somatic impulses that run afoul of normative cultural values—which Freud defined as "the limits that are regarded as normal."[71] Insofar as we humans require one another to sustain our going-on-living, first as dependent infants and later as quasi-independent adults, the individual as such will always remain divided within itself; consequently, all individuals, according to Freud, will suffer psychic conflicts engendered by our social relations. He referred to this condition as "common unhappiness."[72] Insofar as such conflicts remain irreducible for individuals themselves, Simondon argues, they can only vibrate anxiously within us.

Not surprisingly, when Crohn's circumscribed my life as an aspiring individual, I was incredibly anxious. Actually, I was anxious long before my diagnosis. I was one of those children whose limbs shook while sitting still, so I was probably already "explor[ing] the limits of my being" long before my Crohn's diagnosis—indeed, I now consider this anxiety as one of its main causes.[73] So, perhaps my postdiagnosis anxiety simply recapitulated a preexisting condition. Still, whatever anxiety I manifested before Crohn's, the mass quantities of immunosuppressing drugs I ingested after my diagnosis cranked my anxiety up several notches. (As I noted earlier, one of prednisone's well-documented biochemical side effects is anxiety, although I didn't know this at the time.) Needless to say, between the diarrhea and the pills, not to mention the incontinence, adolescence, and proto-queerness, I was an anxious mess. Furthermore, as my mother's son, I had a keenly honed sense of the historical limitations within which I lived, including anti-Semitism, anti-intellectualism, anticommunism, and homophobia, just to name a few. Unfortunately, I had no power to go beyond any of these limits on my own. Hence, anxiety suffused my way of being. It seemed as familiar as the air I breathed.

When I discovered Continuum, I began to sense what the wind person I'd visualized in Naomi's office might really have to offer me. Among its many other gifts, Continuum inspired me to breathe differently. Continuum's movements always involve not just the capacity to intentionally guide breathing—thereby consciously intervening in the tangle of neuromuscular and biochemical processes that breathing entails—but also the possibility of "riding the breath" (much as surfers ride the wave). In learning to ride my breath, I understood that breathing—like wind—demonstrates that from our first breath we are always already participating in complicated processes that take place at much larger (biospheric) and smaller (molecular) scales.[74] After all, even in those moments when we remain most egotistically attached to our individuality, we still have to breathe. Because Continuum uses breathing and sounding, amplified by the group's internal resonance, to score its choreographies, the distinction between "my breath" and the breath of others tends to become increasingly diaphanous, as do our psychosocial investments in being an individual.

As the sense of individuality dilates in the group process of breathing and sounding together, it revises the feeling of what being an individual involves. As a result, the notion that "the (breathing) body" provides a container for "the self" no longer seemed as self-evident as it once had.[75] By undoing the fantasy that as an individual I ought to be able to "contain myself" in the midst of life's torrent of events (including, in my case, the incontinence, the hemorrhaging, the out-of-body experiences and trances, the talking trees, the HIV/AIDS epidemic, etc.), Continuum helped expand my sense of the situation—or perhaps the predicament—within which I sustained myself. It created a transindividual collective that allowed me to revise the terms within which I "put myself into question." This expanded perspective enabled me to reframe some of the psychic problems that persistently plagued my life with Crohn's and, sometimes, even to resolve them. Over many years of joining with others to create inspiring transindividual contexts (inspiring in the most literal sense, since the Latin *inspiro* means "to breathe into"), my persistent anxiety palpably receded, allowing a new, entirely unanticipated, equanimity to emerge, at least from time to time.

Before I discovered Simondon's thinking, I considered such transindividuating moments as part of what I called Continuum's "field effect," which I took to be the most powerful aspect of the practice, although I couldn't really explain why. I knew that when I spent time practicing Continuum in group retreats, I always emerged with a new sense of myself and my place in the world. And over the decades, I discovered that each time I returned to the practice, this experience became more penetrating, even as my sense of self became more diffuse. Adopting Simondon's notion of the transindividual as a frame of reference helped me understand why Continuum had come to mean so much to me. It also enabled me to understand why I increasingly thought of it as my spiritual practice, despite the fact that Emilie and Susan never referred to Continuum using the S-word, as well as the fact that I was raised by devout atheists to reject anything that smacked of the immaterial. Besides, I never much liked the word *spiritual* anyway.

You may have noticed that I have not discussed spirituality in this book thus far, not even when describing my near-death experience, my trances, or my sessions with Naomi, all of which could easily have been rendered as spiritual. This is not an accident. The vagueness of the category "spiritual but not religious," which now brands many American lifestyle-cum-consumer-trends (often represented by personalities like Deepak Chopra, Oprah Winfrey, or Gwyneth Paltrow), has always bugged me. Since I was raised to think of religion as the opiate of the masses, I definitely get the appeal of the not-religious, yet I'd never quite gotten what *spiritual* offers as an alternative way of thinking. Yes, "the spiritual" seems slightly less vague than "the mystery" or "the ineffable" or "the great unknown," whose unspeakableness just obscures the issue; nevertheless, it always appeared to require a bit too much handwaving, crystal gazing, and candle lighting to appeal to my overly critical temperament.[76] However, when Simondon turned to spirituality to invoke the paradoxical or ambiguous nature of the transindividual, he helped me relax my inherited cynicism and put me more at ease with the possibility that things of the spirit might matter.

Simondon begins his reflections on spirituality by clearing the slate. He immediately brackets the Western tendency, which descends from Plato and travels through Christianity before giving birth to the New Age, to associate spirituality with the "other life" rather than this life. Instead, he troubles the opposition between spirit and matter incorporated in this tendency: "Perhaps it must not be said that there is a biological or purely corporeal life, and an other life [*autre vie*], which would be spiritual life in opposition to the former."[77] Rather than overvaluing the transcendent or the eternal, Simondon perceives the instantaneous and the fleeting as essentially spiritual.[78] Hence he advocates what he calls "lived spirituality," by which he means:

> the spirituality of the instant, which does not seek eternity and shines like the light of a gaze only to extinguish itself, [yet it] also really exists. If it didn't also have this luminescent adhesion to the present, this manifestation which gives absolute value to the moment and which consumes sensation, perception, and action within itself, it would not have a spiritual meaning. Spirituality is not an "other life," yet neither is it the same life. It is other and same; it is the meaning of the coherence of the other and the same in a higher [*supérieure*] life. It is the meaning of being as separate and connected, as alone and as a member of the collective; the individuated being is simultaneously on its own and not on its own; it necessarily possesses these two dimensions.[79]

Approaching spirituality as a coincidence of contraries, Simondon evokes it to name the paradox of manifestation not governed by the Aristotelian law of noncontradiction.[80] The "both/and" rhetoric he repeatedly employs here underscores the necessary duplicity of an individuated being, which is both the same as and other than itself. These two putatively opposing dimensions entwined in the individuating individual confound the bifurcating logics (body/soul, matter/form, self/other, subject/object, reality/appearance, inside/outside, individual/milieu, etc.) that underwrite Western metaphysics. Instead of representing one side of a disjunction over and against the other, Simondon proposes that spirituality embraces both; it thereby reveals singularity as always already collective and separation as connected. Furthermore, by perceiving that conjunction depends upon and includes disjunction—and vice versa—Simondon appeals to lived spirituality as a means to overcome the opposition between the one and the many that besets groups which take the individual as their founding premise.

For Simondon, spirituality inheres in both the recognition and the appreciation that individuation can never complete itself at the level of the individual. Instead, the excess of the preindividual that the individual carries along with it can also impel the individuated being to exceed itself toward a more expansive, collective (trans)individuation. Such collective being constitutes a form of spiritual belonging insofar as it not only calls upon the unresolved and irreducible "charge" of the preindividual but also "preserves, respects, and lives within the consciousness of its existence." The immanence of the preindividual within the individual animates the transindividual as a collective individuation that gathers up and "reconnect[s] the separated being."

Needless to say, transindividuation doesn't just happen, it takes practice—sometimes even spiritual practice, using *spiritual* in Simondon's sense. To convoke such a spiritual gathering requires creating a milieu in which individuals can tap into the preindividual aspects of themselves, appreciate the tensions they represent and manifest, and then join with others to resolve them by bringing forth new possibilities for being together. Such convocations have probably been taking place as long as humans have been human—although not necessarily using Simondon's reflexive language. Drumming, dancing, singing, chanting, meditating, and breathing together, for example, can all call forth this aspect of transindividuation insofar as they can all induce an "internal resonance" that gathers disparate elements into transindividuating entities—at least for a time. (Like all individuation, transindividuation is subject to "falling out of phase" and thus to disintegration.) Indeed, most spiritual traditions draw on these kinds of transindividuating technologies in one way or another—that's how they become traditions in the first place. However, since I'd been raised as an atheist, before I started practicing Continuum, all this was news to me.

Although to some Continuum might just seem like one more of those esoteric California retreat programs people love to mock, it never proposed itself as a spiritual endeavor. Thus, it provided the ardent atheist in me with an opportunity to explore the possibilities of transindividuation without having to think about them as spiritual. Given my prejudices at the time, that would have been a major turnoff. Clearly, Continuum might not work for many people—it certainly wouldn't have worked for me before I'd experienced trances and radical healing, conversed with Naomi and discovered psychosynthesis, dipped into tai chi for a few years, and then spent five more years exploring Feldenkrais. And I'm definitely not trying to sell you on it as a privileged path to exploring the possibilities for individual and collective healing. I say *sell* intentionally because, like all the practices I've discussed in this book, Continuum workshops definitely cost money (although they try to offer sliding payment scales to make it affordable to a wider range of participants). Hence, they exclude those for whom such expenses are unaffordable, especially given that no health insurance will cover them—not to mention that the United States doesn't provide universal health insurance in any case. One of the benefits of valuing healing as both a personal and social good might entail expanding medical coverage to all people as well as expanding the range of therapeutic resources that deserve such coverage. Be that as it may, my middle-class resources did enable me to afford these workshops, and they changed my life. Thus, despite this important economic caveat, let me indulge in a brief description of my experience of a Continuum workshop to help you understand why they helped me learn to heal in such profound ways.

No doubt, Susan and Emilie were geniuses at gathering people who had little or no previous connection with each other to move and breathe together for short periods of time, a weekend, a week or two, no more than a month. In workshops of between twenty and forty people that created transindividuating crucibles, we could melt, dissolve, and perhaps resolve some of the psychic and somatic tensions that remained irreducible for each of us separately as individuals. In fact, we came together precisely to recognize and affirm the possibility of healing through community (rather than depending on individual immunity, as Western medicine seemed to suggest we should).[81] In other words, we gathered to participate in a collective process of transindividuation in order to ameliorate problems and anxieties that remained unresolvable on our own.

Continuum workshops have a regular structure. They usually take place in a retreat center, often in a beautiful natural setting—my favorite is Mount Madonna, a yoga ashram at the crest of the Santa Cruz Mountains looking out over the tops of the redwoods down to Monterey Bay. For the first few days of a workshop, as we landed and began to shape our shared space-time container, we grounded ourselves in the group by starting to move and breathe and think and speak and laugh and eat together. Each day we introduced a few cues and themes, perhaps a breathing technique, or a sensory exercise, or a sound, or an intention, or a motif that we would try out for a short while before launching into an improvisational jam for a few hours in which we riffed on these elements, allowing them to amplify and vibrate within us. In each of these "dives" (as we called them) we played together with the elements of a shared movement repertoire, using our bodies as instruments in an ensemble to generate a collective vibe. As we did, we became more and more attuned to sensations, both our own and those called in by the group, cultivating our abilities to express both subtler and wilder tones. By honing our personal capacities, we participated in the group energy with progressively less inhibition from our habituated patterns and gave ourselves over to the transformative process with greater abandon. As a result, we gradually introduced, enhanced, and amplified the "internal resonance" (which Simondon characterized as essential to transindividuation) while we attuned ourselves toward vital possibilities that, even though they might always move through us as traces of the preindividual, remained largely unnoticed and undervalued in our everyday lives.

These first days of a workshop serve as preparation for the main event: the all-nighter (something of a misnomer, since it doesn't involve staying up all night). The all-nighter is an unstructured two- or three-day period in which participants dive into the practice without instruction or prescribed direction, often calling upon and amplifying the cues and motifs introduced in the preceding days, although never limited to these elements. We call this practice an all-nighter because for its duration we agree to move and sound and breathe and sleep in a shared space, creating what we sometimes call a "dream kiva." We intentionally establish this collective dream realm as the container for a transitional phenomenon—to employ the idiom of psychoanalyst Donald Winnicott—by ritually orienting the room around a number of altars that serve as transitional objects to focus our attention and intention according to a range of possible themes or motifs (e.g., elements, ancestors, natural features of the place, mythic characters, the unknown).[82] We also set the temporal boundaries of the all-nighter by ritually opening and closing the event, establishing it as a period during which we attempt to put our habitual attitudes and assumptions about ourselves into abeyance. In so doing, we render this shared space and time sacred—in its etymological sense of set aside, devoted, dedicated—thereby framing the collective experience as an other space-time within this space-time or as an other life within the same life (to recall Simondon's definition of spirituality).[83]

To intensify our focus on the practice and emphasize its status as a time out of time, during the all-nighter we also observe a "verbal fast" that asks us not to use spoken language to communicate; otherwise, we are free to engage, or not, with one another as we wish. By avoiding speech, we intentionally interrupt its highly habitual breath, sound, muscular, and neural patterns—after all, spoken language is audible breath that recurs with recognizable regularities. These repeated series of sounds both consciously and unconsciously overdetermine our ways of being together so that in bracketing them for a period of time, we create intervals in which we can attempt new, nonverbal ways to animate the spaces both within and between us. Moreover, when we interrupt our deep attachments to speech, we change how we attend to both inner and outer acoustics—that is, the voices in our heads as well as other people's voices—which encourages us to innovate nonfamiliar modes of engagement with ourselves and one another through movement, gesture, and nonverbal sound. In other words, it increases our capacities to play, which, as Winnicott emphasizes, underlie both our relational and creative potentials.[84]

Of course, on this playground no one is required to stay with the group, and indeed the only rule in an all-nighter besides trying not to talk is to follow our deepest impulses wherever they take us. Depending on where and when we've gathered, that might include spending large parts of the all-nighter outside, connecting with the ambient surroundings, even as we try to maintain an affective tether to the group back in the room. At Mount Madonna, I often spent hours walking in the redwoods, bathing in their *viriditas*, listening to the streams that dashed down the mountainside to the ocean, following the birds of prey as they soared in spirals over the forest, and contemplating the stars in the night sky (which light pollution renders invisible from my garden at home in Brooklyn). In an all-nighter, time dilates beyond the conventional measuring of contemporary capitalism's 24/7 digital existence.[85] Bracketing our customary temporal and spatial orientations allows us to explore latent possibilities that we always carry with us but that, because of our dominant economic and political value schemata, we mostly disregard as useless—that is, as unworthy ways of spending time. Employing these very simple guidelines, all-nighters open temporal windows onto different value contexts that disrupt our everyday habits of attention and intention. They ask nothing of us apart from investigating the many modes of being present to being alive with other living beings. It turns out that this is asking quite a lot.[86]

By recalling the transindividual impulses that underlie our interests (in the sense of our "between-beings"), the all-nighter establishes a container in which we intentionally investigate moving beyond the specific limitations of our culturally and historically ingrained patterns of being together as humans. The effects of this experimentation are usually profound and require time to unpack and digest. Thus, after we ritually close the all-nighter's temporal window, the last days of a Continuum workshop are devoted to allowing us, as we reclaim spoken language, to report back to the group on our nonverbal adventures during the transitional phenomenon. These narratives frequently reveal moments of radical transformation in which individual participants recall aspects of the group process—perhaps an encounter with another participant, or with an ensemble, or with a dream, or with the world outside—as providing new vistas onto old problems that have dramatically altered how we perceive them as problems. As we do so, resonances between experiences, which might at first have seemed singular, become recognizable as themes that have played throughout the entire group during the workshop. In naming these themes and respecting their significance, we explicitly evoke the transindividuating dimensions of the all-nighter as essential to its transformative effects for each—and all—of us. Given the palpable permutations of this shared spiritual situation, the remainder of our time together involves conjuring and elaborating frameworks for imagining how we will incorporate them into our daily lives.

No doubt this description makes the experience of the all-nighter seem incredibly Californian, or perhaps even worse, New Age. Indeed, even as I offer this account, my inner academic cynic cringes at the apparent romanticism and goopy-aesthetic. It sounds far too woo-woo, I fear. Of course, these days you can find hundreds, if not thousands, of similar testimonials to many such workshops online, each promising a new and different mode of healing. Yet, there is one important distinction between Continuum and these others: it turns out that there is nothing really new about the practices and precepts of Continuum workshops. In fact, they explicitly take their inspiration from an ancient therapeutic technique, Asclepian temple healing, that emerged alongside Hippocratic medicine in the sixth century BCE. The two coexisted for more than a millennium. (As we'll see in a moment, Asclepius was the Greek god of healing, and his temples appeared throughout the Mediterranean basin during the millennium between 500 BCE and 500 CE—when Jesus co-opted Asclepius's healing powers.) Thus, Continuum's Asclepian orientation provides an excellent example of what Foucault called "an insurrection of subjugated knowledges," picking up on a thread of therapeutic possibilities that had largely dropped from awareness for more than fifteen hundred years.

This insurrectionary aspect of Continuum's intent was never subtle. At the beginning of an all-nighter, each time we opened its sacred space-time, Emilie would remind us that the experiences we were about to enter into modeled themselves on Asclepian sanctuaries. Although I knew a bit about the history of medicine before I came to Continuum—I had been reading Foucault for a while by this point and had begun to research the history of immunology— until I heard Emilie refer to Asclepius as an inspiration for the all-nighter, I had never heard his name. In retrospect it seems very telling that I never learned about Asclepius until then, since his symbol actually appears before our eyes with great frequency in everyday life, although very few people would recognize it as such. Indeed, almost every ambulance, pharmacy, or hospital awning sports his icon—as does the cover of this book as well as many of its pages (including this one)—a staff with a single snake entwined around it conventionally known as the rod of Asclepius. Now there's even an emoji: ⚕. (Because Asclepius's legacy remains so obscure, it's often misrepresented with a double snake, which makes it into the caduceus (☤), symbol for the messenger god Hermes, instead.) Although I had seen the familiar symbol myriad times, like most people I had no idea what this common figure referred to, let alone who Asclepius was or what he represented. It's almost as if modern medicine hides its Asclepian heritage in plain sight, flaunting its traces while failing to give them any credit. However, after hearing about the Asclepian dream temples each time I participated in an all-nighter, I realized that if I wanted to know more about what I'd learned from Continuum—and especially about those things that medicine no longer knows—Asclepius definitely warranted a bit more investigation.

While the cult's origins remain a matter of debate, the epicenter for Asclepian healing was undoubtedly the temple—or Asklepion—at Epidaurus founded in the late sixth or early fifth century BCE.[87] From there the cult emigrated, eventually spanning the entire Hellenic and Hellenistic world, first taking root in Athens around 420 BCE. By the time Christianity began its war against the cults it denigrated as pagan in the third and fourth centuries CE, there were around nine hundred Asclepian temples scattered throughout the Hellenic world, the most famous of which, in addition to Epidaurus, Athens, and Rome, appeared in Cos, Pergamum, Tricca, Lebena, Piraeus, Aegae, and Pellene.[88] Many of these sanctuaries were built around springs in which supplicants could bathe before entering the sacred precincts to perform sacrifices at the god's altar. The major temple compounds often included numerous buildings, including peripheral shrines to related gods, as well as stadia, palaestrae, gymnasia, stoai, odea, and theaters, and they were sites of major cultural festivals and rituals as well as athletic competitions. By the imperial Roman period, these buildings often also included baths, guest houses, and other amenities so that Asclepian temples came to function as Hellenistic spas or sanitoria.

Most importantly, an Asklepion included a dormitory or *abaton* in which those seeking the god's healing intercession would sleep amid the god's familiars (snakes and dogs) awaiting dreams in which the god would either heal them or reveal the means of their healing. Here's one version of what the ritual might have been like:

> At most temples dedicated to Asclepius, guests patiently waited until summoned by priests to the abaton for the temple sleep or "*enkoimisis*." The name [*abaton*] meant "impassable place"—a space not to be trespassed, in a word: "pure." Barefoot and dressed in special robes, the purified supplicants stripped of their worldly identity, walked over to this "sacred dormitory" at twilight, where priests assigned each of them a pallet, sometimes stone divans called *klinai* covered with animal skins. After a final prayer, the priests demanded silence, put out the oil lamps, and departed.... Petitioners now anxiously waited for hours—sometimes days—for an epiphany: a healing dream or vision in which Asclepius or his totem animals would appear, touch them, and even face to face proffer advice.[89]

The practice of dream incubation constituted the central rite of Asclepian healing.[90] Having first been "purified" and "stripped of their worldly identity" in a series of collective rituals, the supplicants slept together in the sacred space, inviting the god's dreamed intercession. And dream they did; archaeologists have found more than thirteen hundred stelae thanking the god for healing dreams, and certainly many more have disappeared over the past two millennia. Interpreting these dream records, historians of ancient medicine have traced the historical transformations in the way the god entered dreams in order to heal, ranging from direct healing interventions, to more technical dreams in which the god employed means familiar to Greek medicine, to prescriptive instructions about diet and regime, to symbolic messages that required interpretation with the assistance of the temple's priests.

Whatever form these therapeutic revelations took, however, the stone carvings paid for and left behind by the supplicants attest to many satisfied customers. Furthermore, the fact that these temples not only endured for over a millennium but often significantly developed and expanded their sanctuaries during that time, transforming them into very elaborate pilgrimage sites, indicates that their treatments had considerable appeal as well as success. This success in turn made them targets of the Christ cult that began to assert its dominance, especially after the Roman emperor Constantine converted in the early fourth century CE. As Christians aggressively attacked earlier cultic practices, henceforth described as pagan, they assiduously destroyed the material and imaginary supports for Asclepian temple healing, which disappeared from the Mediterranean region over the next two centuries: "when the god of a new Gospel appeared, [Asclepius] became perhaps his most significant and most powerful antagonist in the spiritual struggle between paganism and Christianity."[91] Thus, despite the widespread cultural and therapeutic value the cult had engendered for over a millennium, after its obliteration by Christianity its insights were suppressed for almost fifteen hundred years.[92]

My initial foray into the history of Asclepian temple healing gave me much material for reflection. It certainly led me to think more seriously about Continuum as picking up the dropped threads of this ancient healing technology and to consider Continuum's Asclepian inspiration as fomenting an uprising of knowledges that had been "disqualified" and "in a way been left to lie fallow, or even kept in the margins," as Foucault framed them.[93] My appreciation for Continuum's conceptual insurgency only increased when I also realized that the rise of Asclepian temple healing was coeval with the invention of Hippocratic medicine around the fifth century BCE and that for the almost one thousand years of Asclepian temple activity, both methods, whether they healed by knowledge or by spirit, not only tolerated one another but often overlapped.[94] Given their initial coexistence, it seems curious that contemporary medicine continues to venerate Hippocrates as the founding father of its particular mode of knowing—if only by requiring each new initiate to ritually intone the Hippocratic oath—while, except for his mysterious glyph, Asclepius has disappeared from the modern therapeutic arena.

In part, this bias reflects the fact that Christians did not attack Hippocrates, who was no threat to their new god, so his followers could continue to practice his knowing ways without opposition.[95] Indeed, we might consider that if Hippocrates personifies medicine's historical orientation toward therapeutic knowledge, then Asclepius might personify our natural tendency toward healing. As Emma and Ludwig Edelstein put it, "Asclepius was the impersonation of the divine healing power; his function was that of giving and preserving health, of relieving from disease." They continue, moreover, "This fact seems proof that his worship, in spite of all its religious aspects was a materialist one, that he was a god of the body rather than the soul. Asclepius played a dominant role in antiquity . . . because of the Greeks' this-worldliness; like them he preferred the visible to the invisible, the life here to the Beyond."[96] Hence Asclepius's absence, as well as the persistent absence of healing itself from modern medical discourses, also betrays a set of assumptions about the ancient possibilities for therapeutic knowledge on which modern medicine continues to rely. As David Morris argues, the difference between how we now regard Hippocrates and Asclepius "suggests a process by which Western medicine sustains its professional, secular, logos-driven enterprise not simply by forgetting its origin, but by erasing or repressing it."[97]

As the first two chapters of *On Learning to Heal* indicate, medicine emerged as such in Greece during the sixth and fifth centuries BCE as a practice that "rules, judges, and cures."[98] It invented two new technologies, diagnosis and prognosis, that defined—and continue to define—knowing as its paramount therapeutic resource. Personified by the figure of Hippocrates, this knowledge practice presented itself as a rational one that rejected recourse to any but natural methods.[99] Underscoring this rationalist belief, the word *physician*, derived from the Greek *phusis* or nature, suggests that, by definition, physicians act on behalf of nature rather than the gods.[100] Indeed, the logical opposition of nature and divine comes into being partly as a result of medicine's own knowledge claims. The emergence of Hippocratic medicine as a unique therapeutic practice exclusively predicated on knowledge helped establish a split within what had previously appeared as a single, albeit polyvalent, mythic world.[101] Thus, in its desire to produce accurate diagnoses and prognoses, if not effective treatments, Hippocratic medicine—insofar as the Hippocratic authors maintained a consistent position on this, which was not always the case—restricted its understanding of nature's divinity to that which conformed with its reason.

In making this distinction, the knowledge practices of Hippocratic medicine corresponded with the developments in philosophy that appeared at exactly the same time.[102] The fundamental conceptual move that philosophy made—and that in turn made it philosophy as we know it—required introducing a disjunction between a world inhabited by the gods and a world inhabited by humans. As a consequence, the latter acquired a uniformity of material causality that the former's unrestricted mutability threatened. The emerging forms of philosophic reason thus rejected the possibility that contraries could coexist, and instead invented contradiction as a mode of disqualification in order to split and thereby purify thought.[103]

Of course, this distinction did not take hold all at once. The coexistence of Hippocratic and Asclepian healing for over a millennium suggests that each logic was allowed its own realm of influence and that neither yet excluded the other from manifesting its own efficacy. However, while this ancient strategy of separate spheres presumed that each recognized the other's specific efficacy, this strategic détente no longer exists. The heirs of Hippocrates—and especially since Claude Bernard transformed the Hippocratic ethos in the middle of the nineteenth century (as discussed in chapter 1)—have increasingly disdained all ambivalence about certain knowledge that Asclepius's lineage represents. While there is much that modern medicine knows it does not know—as the previous chapters underscore—it does not always recognize this not-knowing as a limiting condition on its capacity to know. Thus, following Henri Atlan, we might say: medicine does not know—and indeed often refuses to know— its own ignorance. Instead, medicine continues to disqualify those knowledges that do not revere the laws of identity and noncontradiction, regarding them as unscientific and therefore uninteresting.

The therapeutic powers of modern medicine's bioscientific bio-logic not-withstanding, given how much medicine does not know, it might be helpful to reanimate elements of the Asclepian orientation as a supplement to medical discourse, if only to leave open a conceptual space for the improbable or unexpected events to which medicine often bears witness but fails to accord much value. In other words, the "concept of Asclepius" (as Emma and Ludwig Edelstein put it) might be helpful to medicine in much the same way that Bergson invoked vitalism as a "sort of label affixed to our ignorance, to remind us of it occasionally," that is, as a way of grasping the ignorance that medicine doesn't know it doesn't know. Indeed, this concept might have much to offer medicine as a way to revive the interest in healing that it seems to have forgotten or repressed over the last century and a half.

While we now hold that the efficacy of medicine's knowledge practices relies on its bioscientific underpinnings, the experience of Asclepian temple healing remains largely obscure to us. As Carl Kerényi wryly notes, approaching the god who dwells in the Asklepion "was no visit to a doctor who simply administered medicine: it was an encounter with the naked and immediate event of healing itself."[104] Rather than a trip to the clinic, where we might be subjected to a barrage of tests seeking to determine the biochemical precipitants of our woes, the transformations that took place in the Asclepian temple instead represented "the immediate experience of the divine in the natural miracle of healing."[105] As Kerényi's oxymoron "natural miracle" suggests, the effects of Asclepian healing embrace a confluence of contraries which, although they manifest an internal tension, do not exclude or negate one another.[106]

Asclepian healing reminds us that wherever there is healing, there is epiphany, even when medicine helps to precipitate the ameliorating effect—as my trances first taught me. Unfortunately, what the history of modern medicine has tended to obscure is precisely what Kerényi underscores about Asclepian devotion, that is, that "healing itself is the mystery"—and who can contradict him? By devoting itself exclusively to the therapeutic powers of knowledge, medicine creates a false binary between knowing and not-knowing or, to put it more actively, between knowing and learning. While the power of medicine's knowledge, as well as its power to know, have undoubtedly produced important technologies and treatments that have saved myriad lives—including my own—its claim that its modes of knowing surpass all others seems arrogant, if not short sighted.

Logically speaking, medical knowledge did not require the form of disqualification that medicine introduced at the end of the eighteenth century, when the royal commissions debunked the "imaginary causes" attributed to mesmerism. This exclusionary tactic had much more to do with legitimizing medical authority as the prevailing therapeutic practice insofar as it conformed to the logical precepts of Western rationality—as well as the emerging logics of scientific investigation—than it did with investigating the healing potential that these imaginary causes might produce (which the royal commission admitted they did). In its claimed defense of the unwitting medical consumer who might mistakenly resort to charlatans or quacks, medical authority turned to science to guarantee that its therapies were always the best—as the Carnegie Foundation's president claimed in his introduction to the *Flexner Report*, which transformed the future of medical education in North America.

Alas, modern medicine's use of disqualification to affirm the superiority of its truth claims does not actually contribute to the efficacy of its treatment options. In fact, as has become increasingly evident in fields ranging from psychoneuroimmunology to psychology, placebo studies, and nursing for example, medicine's insistence on establishing knowledge boundaries around which treatments count as therapeutic can unnecessarily restrict our access to potentially effective protocols. In suggesting that the concept of Asclepius might have something important to offer medicine as a way to consider these options—or at least not to exclude them—I am trying to suggest that acknowledging ambiguity as a viable therapeutic attitude does not undermine modern medicine's efficacy and might even enhance its capacity to value healing as part of its practice.

In light of all that I have learned about healing from psychosynthesis, tai chi, ATM, and Continuum, among the many other therapeutic practices I have tried, I am inclined to accept that as important as medicine's resources have been for keeping me alive, they certainly do not exhaust all the effective possibilities on offer. Moreover, the ambiguity of Asclepian healing personally appeals to me as an appropriate attitude toward living with Crohn's disease, given that the best explanation medicine currently offers for Crohn's is that it represents a biological paradox. Insofar as Crohn's continues to be regarded as an autoimmune disease, and autoimmunity is still regarded as the mistaking of self for other, that is, as a self-contradiction, it seems that the disease under whose name I have lived for more than five decades represents a breakdown not only in my identity but in the law of identity per se.[107] That the logic governing the bio-logic of biomedicine cannot redress any of the many diseases currently considered to have autoimmune etiologies might indicate that although Western reason can account for some biological phenomena, it cannot account for them all. Furthermore, it might be worth considering that the rationality that modern medicine takes as its raison d'être has its own limits, limits that descend to it from the inception of medicine's entanglement with Western philosophy almost twenty-five hundred years ago.

In learning about Asclepius, I learned something important about learning to heal. Asclepius came to me first as a way to experience transindividual transformation before I knew anything about either his mythography or the practices of his healing cult. Invoking his name, the Continuum all-nighters gave me a nomenclature to call upon in order to grasp what I felt had been deeply lacking in the ways medicine had taught me to think about myself, insofar as I imagined that I had Crohn's disease. Medicine schooled me in its knowledge practices both by telling me what it thought was wrong with me and then offering prescriptions to treat it. Unfortunately, while they successfully kept me from dying, neither the knowledge nor the treatments ever helped me learn to heal. Moreover, by implying that their treatments were the best if not the only ones that could mitigate my suffering—despite the fact that they actually didn't—they limited my capacity to learn that healing entails learning to live otherwise.

At best, medicine offers to share its knowledge with us, although in doing so it continues to judge and govern us in the service of treating us. However, medicine does not encourage us to learn in the sense that Moshe Feldenkrais emphasized when he asserted that learning always requires us to learn how to learn. Nor does it inspire us to grow in the ways suggested by Hildegard of Bingen's notion that healing resonates with the *viriditas* of plants. Hippocrates, the champion diagnostician, personifies a mode of treatment that confirms the physician as the subject who is supposed to know. More than two thousand years later, we still approach physicians as supplicants who desire that their knowledge can transform our woes. Sometimes our supplications can be answered with an appropriate prescription, procedure, treatment, or surgical intervention, in which case we can appreciate and give thanks for medicine's knowing ways. However, medicine as we know it does not and cannot always fulfill our desires. In such instances, we might benefit from recognizing that what medicine knows does not represent the limits of healing per se. Indeed, such recognition might even provide us with new opportunities to learn to heal.

# Coda

## HEALING WITH COVID, OR

## WHY MEDICINE IS NOT ENOUGH

I opened this book by claiming that the word *healing*, if not the concept, was entirely absent from what (following Paula Treichler's description of HIV/AIDS) we might call the pandemic of signification that COVID-19 catalyzed. This was not strictly true. There was one important exception to this rule: an op-ed that appeared in the *New York Times* on Thanksgiving Day 2020 at the height of the pandemic in the United States. And—although I acknowledge that it gives my inner Lefty queer Jew some trepidation to admit it—that exceptional op-ed was written by the pope. Yet, on reflection, maybe it actually makes sense that it was written by the pope, since for the preceding fifteen hundred years Christ has usurped Asclepius's role as the god of healing. In light of this largely unacknowledged lineage, the pope may in fact be the person closest to being a contemporary apostle of Asclepius—albeit in shepherd's clothes (and with shiny red shoes). Anyway, in his short essay, Pope Francis offered an important counterpoint to the militarized metaphors that have proliferated wildly in both policy and public health discourses about COVID-19.[1]

The pope begins his essay by recounting the story of his falling gravely ill with a rampant lung infection at the age of twenty-one, one that left him with "a sense of how people with COVID-19 feel as they struggle to breathe on a ventilator." Describing how deeply the experience affected him, he wrote: "It changed the way I saw life. For months, I didn't know who I was or whether I would live or die. The doctors had no idea whether I'd make it either." Then, after having the upper lobe of one lung removed, the future pope was left by his physicians to take antibiotics and, they hoped, recover. (Needless to say, I identified here.) Unfortunately, his doctors' prescriptions proved insufficient to the task, and so he remained gravely ill. Fortunately, one of his nurses recognized the doctors' mistake and doubled the dosage of antibiotics, while another nurse noticed that he needed more pain medication and slipped it to him. As a result of the nurses' actions, Francis says he realized not only that modern medicine has real limits but also that, no matter what resources medicine might provide, his life also depended upon his vital connections to others: "They taught me what it is to use science but also to know when to go beyond it to meet particular needs. And the serious illness I lived through taught me to depend on the goodness and wisdom of others."

Taking his own healing seriously, this realization led the pope to advocate an expansive and generous response to COVID-19, lacking in the positions taken by many politicians around the world: "We cannot return to the false securities of the political and economic systems we had before the crisis. We need economies that give to all access to the fruits of creation, to the basic needs of life: to land, lodging, and labor. We need a politics that can integrate and dialogue with the poor, the excluded and the vulnerable, that gives people a say in the decisions that affect their lives. We need to slow down, take stock and design better ways of living together on this earth." While the pope doesn't use the word *healing* here—calling instead for "solidarity"—he certainly gestures in that direction: "Solidarity is more than acts of generosity, important as they are; it is the call to embrace the reality that we are bound by bonds of reciprocity. On this solid foundation we can build a better, different, human future." Healing *with* COVID rather than healing *from* COVID asks us to elaborate these foundational possibilities. To do so, perhaps we need to learn that healing does not belong to us, that we are not its owners, nor are we the owners of our bodies. Instead, learning to heal asks us to reconsider the ways we remain connected to the world and to each other. Because insofar as it tends to take place—even when we're not paying attention to or appreciating that fact—healing can teach us that we always depend on it and on each other in ways that medicine does not (yet?) know. And if and when we learn *that* lesson, then, perhaps, we will also begin to learn how to heal.

# Notes

### A NOTE ON SHIT

1. Deleuze and Guattari, *Anti-Oedipus*, 143.

### OVERTURE. HEALING AS DESIRE AND VALUE

1. Sweet, *God's Hotel*. I thank one of the anonymous readers for Duke University Press for turning me on to Sweet's work.

2. For a concise synthesis of the voluminous literature on humoralism, see Meloni, "Plasticity before Plasticity."

3. Logeion, s.v. "viridis," accessed June 17, 2020, https://logeion.uchicago.edu/viridis. On *viriditas* in Hildegard's mystical texts, see Marder, "On the Vegetal Verge."

4. Sweet, *God's Hotel*, 97; Sweet, "Hildegard of Bingen"; Logeion, s.v. "viriditas," accessed June 17, 2020, https://logeion.uchicago.edu/viriditas.

5. Sweet, *Rooted in the Earth*, 152–54.

6. Sweet, *God's Hotel*, 97.

7. Sweet, *God's Hotel*, 105–6.

8. Sweet, *God's Hotel*, 107.

9. Sweet, *Slow Medicine*.

10. Sweet, *God's Hotel*, 111.

11. Nietzsche, *Will to Power*, 380.

12. *Conatus* is a nominal form of the Latin verb *conor*, meaning to undertake, endeavor, attempt, try, venture, seek, aim, make an effort, begin. Logeion, s.v. "conor," accessed May 26, 2020, https://logeion.uchicago.edu/conor. It has been used for over two thousand years to try to conceptualize the self-persistence of both animate and inanimate beings.

13. Spinoza, *Ethics*, vol. 3, prop. 6 and 7, 283.

14. Spinoza, *Ethics*, vol. 3, preface. "Most of those who have written about the emotions [*affectibus*] and human conduct seem to be dealing not with natural phenomena that follow the common laws of Nature but with phenomena outside Nature. They appear to go so far as to conceive man in Nature as a kingdom within a kingdom" (277).

15. Vernadsky, *Biosphere*.

16. Bergson, *Creative Evolution*, 83. I return to Bergson's ideas in chapter 1.

17. Logeion, s.v. "valere," accessed May 30, 2020, https://logeion.uchicago.edu/valere.

18. Going-on-living is not necessarily always a paramount value, but if it is not, then the conditions of life can start to tend toward death.

19. Canguilhem, "Health," 472.

20. Whitehead, *Function of Reason*, 5.

21. Atlan, "Knowledge of Ignorance," 386.

22. While a far from uncontested category, biomedicine generally refers to the confluence of three trends that occurred in the wake of World War II: the tendency of the life sciences to focus inquiry at the level of molecules, the adoption of mathematical and especially computer-based modeling, and the linking of clinical practice to laboratory experimentation. Gaudillière, *Inventer la biomédicine*; Clarke et al., "Biomedicalization."

23. Roosth, *Synthetic*.

24. Michel Foucault, "Introduction," in Canguilhem, *Normal and the Pathological*, 21.

25. Atlan, "Knowledge of Ignorance," 388.

26. Atlan, "Knowledge of Ignorance," 389.

27. Deny, "Evidence-Based Medicine"; Derkatch, "Method as Argument."

28. Atlan, "Knowledge of Ignorance," 385.

29. Brier, *Infectious Ideas*.

30. For example, see Patton, *Sex and Germs*; Treichler, "AIDS, Homophobia, and Biomedical Discourse"; Watney, *Policing Desire*; Epstein, *Impure Science*.

31. Ehrenreich and English, *Witches, Midwives, and Nurses*; Fett, *Working Cures*; Savitt, *Race and Medicine*; Breslaw, *Lotions, Potions, Pills and Magic*.

32. Although we should also recognize that modern medicine often doesn't know why its treatments work; for example, millions of prescriptions for selective serotonin reuptake inhibitors (SSRIs) have been filled to treat depression, despite the fact that the biochemistry of affect and mood remain only vaguely understood.

33. The refrain "poison, slash, burn" accompanies the choreography of *Still/Here*, a 1994 work by Bill T. Jones based on interviews with people who were facing life-threatening illnesses. Bill T. Jones, *Still/Here*, 1994, New York Live Arts, https://newyorklivearts.org /repertory/stillhere/.

34. I was recently reminded of this during a presurgical appointment with the chief orthopedic surgeon at a famous New York hospital to discuss an upcoming hip replacement. After he finished explaining in exquisite technical detail the intricate dynamics of the operation and extolling the wonders of the titanium prosthetics he planned to implant in my body, I casually asked him if he had any suggestions about healing after the procedure. His reply was classic: "No," he said, "just go home, take the pain killers, and do the physical therapy exercises."

35. One of the first published conference proceedings on the topic defines compliance as "the extent to which the patient's behavior (in terms of taking medications, following diets, or executing other life-style changes) coincides with clinical prescription." Haynes and Sackett, *Compliance with Therapeutic Regimes*, 1. For an extended critique of the disciplinary effects of compliance as a strategy of medical governance, see Kane, *Pleasure*

*Consuming Medicine*. For a reflection on the idiom of compliance and some alternatives, see Fawcett, "Thoughts about Meanings of Compliance." As of June 7, 2021, Medline lists over 150,000 entries on the topic heading "compliance."

36. Although he does not refer to toilet training as such—instead simply demurring that he could elaborate innumerable facts about the "hygiene of natural needs"—Marcel Mauss underscores the cultural variation in all such techniques of the body. He argues that "these [corporeal] techniques are the human norms of human training [*dressage*]. These techniques which we apply to animals, humans voluntarily apply to themselves and their children. The latter are probably the first to have been thus trained [*dresser*]—before all other animals, which first had to be domesticated [*apprivoiser*]." Mauss, "Les techniques des corps," 16.

37. As early as 1936, the eminent medical historian Henry Sigerist proclaimed, "Medicine is not a branch of science, and it will never be. If medicine is a science, then it is a social science." Sigerist, "History of Medicine," 5.

38. In his inaugural lecture at the Collège de France, Michel Foucault elaborates this strategy of disqualification and boundary maintenance. He attributes the phrase "in the true" (*dans le vrai*) to Georges Canguilhem. Foucault, "Discourse on Language," 224.

39. Science and technology studies has invested a lot of effort in detailing such boundary maintenance procedures. See Gieryn, "Boundary-Work"; Gieryn, *Cultural Boundaries of Science*; Bazerman, *Shaping Written Knowledge*. In relation to bioscience, see Meyers, *Writing Biology*.

40. Foucault, *Society Must Be Defended*, 7.

41. The National Center for Complementary and Integrative Health was founded in 1991 as the Office of Alternative Medicine. It changed its name to the National Center for Complementary and Alternative Medicine in 1998 and to its current name in 2014. As these renamings indicate, the relation between "proper" medicine and its "others" is a shifting one. In any case, the NCCIH is the least funded of the National Institutes of Health and has been subject to constant criticism for its methods and goals ever since it was founded.

42. Foucault, *Society Must Be Defended*, 8.

CHAPTER ONE. HEALING TENDENCIES

1. Neuburger, *Doctrine of the Healing Power*; Canguilhem, "Idea of Nature."

2. Normandin and Wolfe, *Vitalism and the Scientific Image*.

3. I'm happy to report that new forms of vitalism are emerging. Monica Greco's work represents one of the best examples. See Greco, "On the Art of Life"; Greco, "On Illness and Value."

4. Abram, "Mechanical and the Organic," 67.

5. Descartes, *Meditations on First Philosophy*, 58. Descartes had an abiding interest in health and illness—including if not especially his own—and in his correspondence professed a less rigid notion of the body. Shapin, "Descartes the Doctor."

6. Abram argues that this recentering of God as both lawmaker and animating force made mechanism more appealing to Church authorities than the preceding Renaissance worldview, which could tend toward heresy, as the execution of Giordano Bruno attests: "The mechanical philosophy became a central facet of the scientific worldview precisely

because it implied the existence of a maker (a divine interpreter) and thus made possible an alliance between science and the Church." Abram, "Mechanical and the Organic," 67.

7. For an overview of these changes in mechanism, see Craver and Tabery, "Mechanisms in Science."

8. The word *homeostasis* was coined in 1926 by Walter Canon in "Physiological Regulation of Normal States."

9. Bernard, *Principes de médecine expérimentale*, 11.

10. In *Life Death*, his 1976 seminar course at the École Normale Supérieur, Jacques Derrida takes up the ways biological discourses embed textual metaphors and models in their attempts to inscribe life within the domain of science.

11. Canguilhem, *Études d'histoire et de philosophie*, 131.

12. Although the contemporary interest in non-Western practices, like traditional Chinese medicine or Ayurvedic medicine, suggests a renewed popular appreciation for some of its premises.

13. *Vaccine* (from the Latin *vacca* for cow) was initially used by Edward Jenner in the late eighteenth century to refer to the use of cowpox, which produced mild symptoms, as a prophylactic against the more serious smallpox. At the end of the nineteenth century, Pasteur strategically appropriated Jenner's specific term as a generic concept in order to promote the attenuated cultures he produced in his lab by nominally associating them with Jenner's famous discovery.

14. Pelis, "Prophet for Profit"; Brisou, "Saigon, Nha-Trang, Hanoi"; Moulin, "Patriarchal Science"; Guénel, "Creation of the First Overseas Pasteur Institute."

15. Nietzsche made a similar point when he admonished us to recall that we are "artistically creating subjects." Nietzsche, "On Truth and Non-truth."

16. Bergson, *Creative Evolution*, 194.

17. Bergson, *Creative Evolution*, 15: "The systems science deals with are, in fact, in an instantaneous present that is always being renewed; such systems are never in that real, concrete duration in which the past remains bound up with the present. . . . In short, *the world that the mathematician deals with is a world that dies and is born at every instant.*"

18. Bergson, *Creative Evolution*, 294. For example, while Darwinism assumed, and still assumes, a reductionist basis for evolutionary development, proposing that potentially infinite, minute, random changes in genetic material (mostly achieved through mutation, horizontal gene transfer, or "random drift") can explain macroscopic changes in species—a dogma that is increasingly challenged by bioscience itself—it still offers no robust account of how or why such changes occur when they occur, let alone why and how they occur in the ways they occur.

19. Bergson, *Creative Evolution*, 285.

20. Bergson, *Creative Evolution*, 139.

21. Bergson, *Creative Evolution*, 20. Fifty years later, following Bergson's lead, another great French philosopher of life, Georges Canguilhem, who was also a doctor, put it slightly more positively: "Vitalism is the expression of the confidence the living being has in life, of the self-identity of life within the living human being conscious of living." Canguilheim, *Knowledge of Life*, 62.

22. Bergson, *Creative Mind*, 246.

23. Lacan, *Les quatre concepts fondamenteaux*, 210–11. For a Lacanian reading of medical authority, see Clavreul, *L'ordre médical*.

24. Suzuki, *Zen Mind, Beginner's Mind*.

25. Petryna, *When Experiments Travel*.

26. Dumit, *Drugs for Life*.

27. Hacking, *Taming of Chance*. Once invented, the calculus of probability was immediately used to assess the value of variolization (inoculation with live smallpox) in relation to its known risk (getting smallpox).

28. The French sociologist of science Bruno Latour characterizes this shift as "the entirely psychological shift *from uncertainty to probability*, a passage facilitated, amplified, justified, and formatted by the spread of accounting instruments and calculating devices." Latour and Lépinay, *Science of Passionate Interests*, 63.

29. Turner, *Radical Remission*.

30. Nagel, *View from Nowhere*.

31. Logeion, s.v. "experior," accessed February 5, 2019, https://logeion.uchicago.edu/experior; Logeion, s.v. "πεıρα," accessed February 5, 2019, https://logeion.uchicago.edu/πεıρα; Logeion, s.v. "περάω," accessed February 5, 2019, https://logeion.uchicago.edu/περάω.

32. Bergson, *Creative Evolution*, 142.

33. Carel, *Illness*.

34. Kleinman, *Illness Narratives*.

35. Following the population model of disease, for the last fifty years medicine has increasingly relied on a new category, "risk," that now in itself serves as a major pretext for medical intervention. Dumit, *Drugs for Life*, describes the shift in biomedicine's therapeutic orientation (as mediated by the pharmaceutical industry) through which risk rather than the manifest symptoms of disease became the basis for preemptive treatments.

36. Canguilhem, *Normal and the Pathological*, 121.

37. Susan Sontag eloquently made this point in her books *Illness as Metaphor* and *AIDS and Its Metaphors*.

38. Treichler, *How to Have Theory*.

39. Logeion, s.v. "valere," accessed February 6, 2019, https://logeion.uchicago.edu /valere.

40. O'Rourke, *Invisible Kingdom*.

41. This could change if bioscientific understandings of brain function ever progress that far, but personally I'm not holding my breath.

42. Frank, *At the Will of the Body*, 45.

43. Logeion, s.v. "tendere," accessed February 5, 2019, https://logeion.uchicago.edu /tendere.

44. This reading of Bergson is indebted to Bernard Stiegler's work and especially his fondness for spirals.

45. Derrida, *Life Death*.

46. "Open up a Few Corpses" is a chapter title in Foucault, *Birth of the Clinic*. Foucault adopts the idiom from the work of the early pathological anatomist Marie-Francois-Xavier Bichat, who used the phrase in his book *Recherches physiologique*.

47. Canguilhem, "Une pédagogie de guérison," 26.

48. Logeion, s.v. "legere," accessed February 5, 2019, https://logeion.uchicago.edu /legere.

49. In *Slow Medicine*, the physician and historian of medicine Victoria Sweet describes the ways that the dominant training in and practice of modern medicine undermine the ethos of care.

50. OED Online, s.v. "care," n. 1, March 2020, Oxford University Press, https://www -oed-com.proxy.libraries.rutgers.edu/view/Entry/27899. A similar tension lies in the Latin *cura*, meaning trouble, care, attention, pains, industry, diligence, exertion, from which *cure* arises: Logeion, s.v. "cura," accessed May 9, 2020, https://logeion.uchicago .edu/cura.

51. Winnicott, "Psychosomatic Illness," 510.

52. Frank, *At the Will of the Body*, 50, emphasis added.

53. From Deleuze's 1986 Paris-VIII seminar on Foucault. Quoted in Dosse, *Gilles Deleuze and Félix Guattari*, 309.

54. Foucault, "Polemics, Politics, and Problematizations."

55. Foucault, "Impossible Prison," 277. Also see Foucault, *Politics of Truth*, 59ff.

56. Foucault, "Truth, Power and Self," 10.

57. In his later work, whether or not one wants to consider him in this way, Foucault adopted a term from Greek antiquity, *psychagogy*, that he contrasted to its more familiar twin, *pedagogy*, to refer to this kind of life-changing practice. See Cohen, "Live Thinking."

58. On why Foucault is my favorite thinker, see Ardele Lister's film *Flower/Power*, 2010, https://ardelelister.com/flower-power.

59. Foucault, *Birth of the Clinic*, 8.

60. Foucault, *Birth of the Clinic*, 136, 155.

61. Abou Farman describes this bodily inscription of death as an existential sign characteristic of the "secular eschatology" that emerged in eighteenth-century Europe. See Farman, *On Not Dying*, 1–78.

62. Foucault, *Les machines à guérir*.

63. Foucault, *Birth of the Clinic*, 146.

64. Philosopher Ian Hacking refers to this kind of productive naming as "dynamic nominalism." Hacking, *Historical Ontology*.

CHAPTER TWO. WE ARE MORE COMPLICATED THAN WE KNOW

1. Kronos famously devoured his own offspring to forestall a prophecy that one of them would overthrow him, not knowing that Zeus's mother Rhea had deceived him by delivering up a rock wrapped in swaddling clothes instead. Zeus eventually fulfilled the prophecy by giving Kronos an emetic that caused him to vomit up Zeus's siblings, who joined Zeus in a war that defeated the Titans and installed the Olympian pantheon. Needless to say, the central dyspeptic event of this epic tale makes it a great allegory for chronic digestive disorders.

2. Dijck, *Transparent Body*; Slatman, "Transparent Bodies"; Kevles, *Naked to the Bone*.

3. The famous formulation of this pharmacological paradox appears in Derrida, "Plato's Pharmacy."

4. "A quantitative difference matters insofar as it takes on a vital value for the living being, be it the patient or the physician." Han and Das, "Introduction," 16.

5. Recent bioscientific explorations have troubled the scriptural assumptions that underwrote the classic dogma of DNA by arguing that naked DNA alone does not express itself in the structures and functions of cells, but rather involves complex processes that include developmental and environmental inputs. In other words, DNA no longer appears to contain the entire text of the "book of life." Derrida reads Nobel Prize winner François Jacob's *The Logic of Life* in order to interrogate biology's metaphoric recruitment of "text" to underwrite this central dogma. Derrida, *Life Death*.

6. Foucault, "Truth and Juridical Forms," 9.

7. Metaphor, from the Greek *meta* + *phora*, to carry across, requires that the elements brought into play—and metaphor is, after all, a play on words—remain irreducible to one another. If there is no gap or tension between them, metaphor collapses into either cliché or tautology. "My love is like a rose" works metaphorically; "my rose is like a flower" does not. Nietzsche, "On Truth and Non-truth." On metaphor in bioscience, see Cohen, *A Body Worth Defending*, 33–38.

8. Van der Eijk, *Medicine and Philosophy*. "Greek doctors . . . had to impress their audiences, to persuade them of their competence and authority, to attract customers and to reassure them that they were much better off with them than their rivals" (30).

9. Logeion, s.v. "θεραπεύω," accessed February 3, 2019, https://logeion.uchicago.edu /θεραπεύω.

10. Logeion, s.v. "prognosis," accessed February 15, 2019, https://logeion.uchicago.edu /prognosis.

11. Jones, *Hippocrates II*, 8–9.

12. Logeion, s.v. "κρίσις," accessed January 15, 2021, https://logeion.uchicago.edu /κρίσις.

13. Logeion, s.v. "rego," accessed February 14, 2019, https://logeion.uchicago.edu/rego; Logeion, s.v. "δίαιτα," accessed February 14, 2019, https://logeion.uchicago.edu/δίαιτα.

14. Benveniste, "La doctrine médicale des Indo-Européens."

15. Benveniste, "La doctrine médicale des Indo-Européens," 7.

16. Foucault, "Subject and Power," 790.

17. As the *Oxford English Dictionary* indicates, a circle of meaning exists between medicine and its "premeditated" practice: *premeditate* derives from the Latin *praemeditārī* ("to contemplate or consider in advance"), which itself derives from *prae-* + *meditārī* ("meditate"), and *meditārī* derives from *med-*. Moreover, as Benveniste corroborates, *med-* provides the base that engenders the classical Latin adjective and noun *medicus*, which derives in turn from the verb *medērī*: "to heal, to remedy, relieve, amend, correct, restore." So the premeditation of medicine appears deeply entangled in its etymological roots.

18. In March 2019, the average retail price for a two-pen package of Humira was around $9,102; for Remicade, a five-vial package goes for around $7,125; for Cosentyx, a two-pen package retails for $9,149 (see GoodRx, https://www.goodrx.com/humira, https://www.goodrx.com/remicade, https://www.goodrx.com/cosentyx [all accessed July 24, 2021]). Pharmaceutical companies do offer discounts and coupons, however. On the power of pharmaceutical ads and PR in general, see Dumit, *Drugs for Life*.

19. Molodecky et al., "Increasing Incidence and Prevalence." On the role of pharmaceutical advertising in the dissemination of disease categories, see Dumit, *Drugs for Life*.

20. Orrego and Quintana, "Darwin's Illness"; Paulley, "Death of Albert Prince Consort."

21. Crohn, Ginzburg, and Oppenheimer, "Regional Ileitis." Crohn himself didn't use the idiom "Crohn's disease," referring instead first to "terminal ileitis" and then, because of the unfortunate double connotations of "terminal" (i.e., end of the ileum and end of life), to "regional ileitis."

22. Fowler, *A Dictionary of Practical Medicine*, 883–84.

23. Alas, this was wishful thinking on Dr. Crohn's part. Although up to 80 percent of those diagnosed with Crohn's will undergo surgery at some point, it is not considered a "complete cure," as relapses after surgery are common. A review article on Crohn's disease repeatedly insists that "there is no cure." Cosnes et al., "Epidemiology and Natural History."

24. Crohn and Janowitz, "Reflections on Regional Ileitis."

25. Furness, *Enteric Nervous System*. For a popular and nicely illustrated explication that became "an instant New York Times Best Seller" (as advertised on Amazon), see Enders, *Gut*.

26. Mayer, "Gut Feelings."

27. "The GI tract represents a direct portal to the molecular universe, and the unique juxtaposition of its nervous and immune systems suggests a vital role for neuro-immune interactions in the gut." Yoo and Masmanian, "Enteric Network."

28. Øyri, Műzes, and Sipos, "Dysbiotic Gut Microbiome."

29. Root-Bernstein, "Antigenic Complementarity," 274.

30. Pastorelli et al., "Central Role of the Gut."

31. Fiocchi, "Inflammatory Bowel Disease Pathogenesis."

32. Glocker and Grimbacher, "Inflammatory Bowel Disease"; Behr, Divangahi, and Lalande, "What's in a Name?"; Folwaczny, Glas, and Torok, "Crohn's Disease."

33. McDermott and Aksentijevich, "Autoinflammatory Syndromes."

34. Burnet, *Clonal Selection Theory*; Burnet, *Self and Not-Self*.

35. On the paradox of autoimmunity in general, see Cohen, "Self, Not-Self."

36. Paul Ehrlich, in *Studies in Immunity*, writes: "One might be justified in speaking of a 'horror autotoxicus' of the organism. These contrivances are naturally of the highest importance for the existence of the individual. During the individual's life, even under physiological though especially under pathological conditions, the absorption of all material of its own body can and must occur very frequently. The formation of tissue autotoxins would therefore constitute a danger threatening the organism more frequently and much more severely than all exogenous injuries" (82–83). For a consideration of how Ehrlich's dogma gave way to the study of autoimmune disease, see Silverstein, "Horror Autotoxicus versus Autoimmunity."

37. Five phenomena—autoimmunity, cancer, pregnancy, host-versus-graft disease, and commensal bacteria—persistently defy the self/not-self paradigm. A few countertheories have emerged over the past seventy-five years, most convincingly Polly Matzinger's "danger theory," but none have established themselves as robust. Matzinger, "Evolution of the Danger Theory"; Matzinger, "Friendly and Dangerous Signals."

38. Chamberlin and Naser, "Integrating Theories of the Etiology."

39. Plevy and Targan, "Future Therapeutic Approaches."

40. Prednisone was first isolated and identified in 1950 and became commercially viable in 1955, trademarked as Meticorten. It began to be prescribed for Crohn's in the late 1950s, with the first clinical assessment of that use appearing in the mid-1960s. Jones and Lennard-Jones, "Corticosteroids and Corticotrophin."

41. Logeion, s.v. "φάρμακον," accessed February 24, 2019, https://logeion.uchicago .edu/φάρμακον; and Logeion, s.v. "φαρμακός," accessed February 24, 2019, https:// logeion.uchicago.edu/φαρμακός. Jacques Derrida elaborates upon these antithetical meanings in "Plato's Pharmacy."

42. As long ago as 1977, five years after I was diagnosed, George Engle diagnosed this "crisis" in contemporary medicine: "Medicine's crisis stems from the logical inference that since 'disease' is defined in terms of somatic parameters, physicians need not be concerned with psychosocial issues which lie outside medicine's responsibility and authority." Engel, "Need for a New Medical Model."

43. An interdisciplinary field of bioscience, psychoneuroimmunology, also called psychoendoneuroimmunology or psychoneuroendocrinoimmunology, has emerged precisely to encompass these types of affecting variables—though sadly with limited impact on clinical practice in gastroenterology.

44. Foucault, "Preface to the History of Sexuality," 335.

45. Stengers, "Doctor and the Charlatan," 129.

46. As another feminist philosopher of science, Donna Haraway, reminds us, "Life is a window of vulnerability. It seems a mistake to close it." Haraway, "Biopolitics of Postmodern Bodies," 224.

47. On the challenges of receiving a useful diagnosis while living with a chronic illness, see O'Rourke, *Invisible Kingdom*.

48. I'm not sure that epidemiology still supports this correlation; however, an article in *PLoS Genetics* indicates that it still has some currency. Kenny et al., "A Genome-wide Scan."

49. Whitehead, *Function of Reason*, 64.

50. While there is still no explanation for why both humans and plants produce cannabinoids, there is now evidence that endogenous human cannabinoids are expressed in breast milk and may function in important ways in both pre- and postnatal neurological development as well as stimulating the sucking reflex, among others, which may explain why some people get the munchies when they get stoned. Gaitán et al., "Endocannabinoid Metabolome Characterization"; Fride, "Endocannabinoid-CB(1) Receptor System." Thanks to Polly Matzinger for pointing out this connection.

51. The first reported cases of what we now call AIDS appeared in the *Morbidity and Mortality Weekly Report* in June 1982—the month I was admitted to Stanford Hospital. The acronym AIDS appeared in September 1982, the month I was released from the hospital. CDC, "A Cluster of Kaposi's Sarcoma."

52. The racial and class disparities in medical coverage in the United States are widely documented. In the wake of COVID-19, much of the media coverage about "vaccine hesitancy" among African Americans underscores the lasting effects of the Tuskegee Institute

syphilis study on attitudes toward clinical medicine. Similarly, racial disparities in care during childbirth (recently personified by tennis star Serena Williams, a multimillionaire married to a billionaire who nonetheless was subject to postnatal neglect) as well as pain management inform attitudes toward clinical practices.

CHAPTER THREE. WE ARE MORE IMAGINATIVE THAN WE THINK

1. Rachel Remen, interview by Charlie Rose, *The Power of Questions*, June 29, 2001, https://charlierose.com/videos/3164.

2. For an overview, see the description posted by the Remen Institute for the Study of Health and Illness (RISHI), accessed July 7, 2021, https://rishiprograms.org/healers-art/.

3. Bill Moyers, "Wounded Healers," *Healing and the Mind*, February 24, 1993, https://billmoyers.com/content/wounded-healers/.

4. In *On Kissing, Tickling and Being Bored*, Adam Phillips makes a parallel point: "As a form of treatment psychoanalysis is a conversation that enables them to understand what stops them from having the kinds of conversations they want, and how they have come to believe these particular conversations are worth wanting. . . . Psychoanalysis is a conversation that helps people get back on track" (6).

5. During one of our first sessions, Naomi recommended I read Dossey, *Space, Time, and Medicine*. Dossey's book troubles modern medicine's foundations in Newtonian physics and wonders how a more post-Newtonian perspective might change the ways that medicine understands the human body.

6. Talal Asad provides a pithy description of biomedicine: "an institutionalized practical knowledge that presents itself as rational and progressive, and sometimes as an epistemological model that can be opposed to theological definitions and explanations of unwellness." Asad, "Thinking about the Secular Body," 338. Obviously, this market dominance is sustained by insurance reimbursements, both public and private. However, according to a recent study of the topic, Americans pay almost as much out of pocket for "alternative and complementary" therapies as for orthodox medical ones. Of course, given the insurance reimbursements, the spending on the latter massively exceeds the former. Nahin, Barnes, and Stussman, "Expenditures on Complementary Health Approaches," 1–6.

7. Starr, *Social Transformation of American Medicine*.

8. The US Supreme Court upheld the constitutionality of such laws in 1889, affirming the legal principle that "the State, in the exercise of its power to provide for the general welfare of its people, may exact from parties before they can practice medicine a degree of skill and learning in that profession upon which the community employing their services may confidently rely, and, to ascertain whether they have such qualifications, require them to obtain a certificate or license from a board or other authority competent to judge in that respect." Dent v. West Virginia, 129 US 114. The Court extended this ruling in Hawker v. New York, 170 US 189 (1898), when a doctor convicted of performing abortions in 1873 was barred from further medical practice due to his prior criminal conviction.

9. Savitt, *Race and Medicine*, 224–36.

10. Starr, *Social Transformation of American Medicine*, 123.

11. Flexner, *Medical Education in the United States*.

12. See, for example, recent articles collated by Science Direct, accessed November 1, 2019, https://www.sciencedirect.com/topics/medicine-and-dentistry/flexner-report.

13. As Paul Starr avers, "The mere existence of competing parties in medicine was a standing rebuke to the claims of orthodoxy to represent a science." Starr, *Social Transformation of American Medicine*, 99.

14. Flexner, *Medical Education in the United States*, x, emphasis added.

15. Starr points out that the *Flexner Report* guided philanthropy, not only of the Carnegie Foundation but of other major foundations, including the Rockefeller Foundation: "The report was a manifesto of a program that by 1936 guided $91 million from the Rockefeller's General Education Board (plus millions more from other foundations) to a select group of medical schools. . . . These policies determined not so much which institutions would survive as which would dominate, how they would be run, and what ideals would prevail." Starr, *Social Transformation of American Medicine*, 121.

16. The latter pedagogy was just as important as the former, if the former was to garner the credit and compensation commensurate with its professional profile—although, of course, always for the public good and the health of the nation: "The interests of the general public have been so generally lost sight of in this matter that the public has in large measure forgot that it has any interests to protect. And yet in no other way does education touch more closely the individual than in the quality of the medical training which institutions of the country provide. Not only the personal well-being of each citizen, but national, state and municipal sanitation rests upon the quality of training which the medical graduate has received. The interest of the public is to have well-trained practitioners in sufficient number for the needs of society." Flexner, *American College*, xvi.

17. Flexner, *Medical Education in the United States*, 25, emphasis added.

18. Flexner, *Medical Education in the United States*, 25.

19. Flexner, *Medical Education in the United States*, 24.

20. Mazumdar, *Species and Specificity*.

21. Farley, "Parasites and the Germ Theory"; Koch, "Etiology of Anthrax"; Pasteur, "Sur les maladies virulentes."

22. The word *vaccine*, from the Latin *vacca* for cow, was used by Edward Jenner at the turn of the nineteenth century to describe his technique for inoculating humans with the relatively benign matter from cowpox to induce resistance to infections by the much more dangerous smallpox. Jenner's innovation was widely heralded as the most significant medical advance against contagious disease before germ theory validated the notion that epidemic diseases were contagions. Precisely because it carried this popular significance as a great medical leap forward, Pasteur appropriated Jenner's term *vaccine* to brand his new technique, even though his experiments involved chickens and not cows. Needless to say, contemporary vaccines have entirely lost their initial bovine connotations. Geison, *Private Science of Louis Pasteur*; Latour, *Pasteurization of France*.

23. The latest iterations of which, of course, now include vaccines that induce resistance to SARS-CoV-2. However, the technologies incorporated in the SARS-CoV-2 vaccines do not recapitulate the killed or attenuated pathogen models that followed Pasteur's innovations. Rather, they are complex technological products that utilize small segments of viral genetic material that are then manipulated in a variety of ways and packaged in

envelopes that allow them to be injected into the human body. Kyriakidis et al., "SARS-CoV-2 Vaccines Strategies."

24. Metchnikoff was led to his insight by his interest in the evolutionary conservation of traits. He perceived the amoeboid cells he named "macrophages" (literally, "big eaters") as repurposing the mechanisms that the single-celled organisms used to digest food to break down invasive bacteria.

25. Before Metchnikoff introduced immunity-as-host-defense in 1883, for over two thousand years immunity had represented an exclusively political and legal premise. Within the Hippocratic/Galenic framework—based on supporting and encouraging the *vis medicatrix naturae*—immunity actually made no sense medically because its legal meaning appeared to be a non sequitur. In legal terms, if you are immune, you don't need to defend yourself, and if you must defend yourself, you're not immune. In fact, in order for immunity to serve as the conceptual crux for germ theory's new bio-logic, Metchnikoff had to completely revise its prior juridico-political significance. After Metchnikoff, (biological) immunity no longer preempted the need for (legal) defense but instead came to represent the way that organisms actively defend themselves against infectious pathogens: that is, Metchnikoff affirmed not that immunity precludes the need for defense, but that biological immunity *is* host defense. On the lasting importance of Bernard's and Metchnikoff's innovations, see Cohen, *A Body Worth Defending*.

26. Canguilhem, "Idea of Nature," 29.

27. Metchnikoff, "Yeast Disease of Daphnia." The original appeared in *Archiv für pathologische Anatomie und Physiologie* 96 (1884): 178–93.

28. While Metchnikoff introduced the idea of immunity as host defense in the late nineteenth century, the concept of the "immune system" did not begin to signify a "diffuse organ ... diffused throughout the entire body" until 1973, when Niels Jerne described it as such in his famous *Scientific American* article. Prior to 1970, the phrase "immune system" rarely appears in medical literature, and when it does, it has a variety of inconsistent meanings. Jerne, "Immune System."

29. Not surprisingly, not long after Metchnikoff published his findings, the scientifically and entrepreneurially savvy Pasteur brought him to the institute he had recently founded in Paris, where Metchnikoff (who won the Nobel Prize in Medicine in 1908) remained ensconced for the rest of his life.

30. Flexner, *Medical Education in the United States*, 24–25.

31. For a quick overview of the complexities that "causality" incorporates, see Hoefer, "Causal Determinism."

32. The idea that causes could be specific dominated biomedical thinking well into the middle of the twentieth century and provided the model for early thinking about genetic determinism:

> In immunology, bacteriology, enzymology, and taxonomy ... specificity served as a laboratory tool for ordering, predicting, and sometimes measuring activities and relations (cross-reactivities) of molecules, organisms, and species or "races." ... More importantly, specificity was primarily a *biological* concept, signifying animate phenomena, processes, and characteristics. As such, specificity related form to

function by representing life within a three-dimensional biological space (or four-dimensional, when including ontogeny's time arrow). Within the epistemic, technical, and disciplinary configurations linking genes, antibodies, enzymes, organismic growth, and animal taxonomy, biological and chemical specificities were central. They accounted, often in material terms and concrete methods, for the myriad of spatial and temporal events from reproduction, fertilization, embryogenesis, maturation, to speciation; specificities dictated and governed the successive cycles of life. Kay, *Who Wrote the Book?*, 46.

33. The story of Koch's quest for the cause of cholera provides one of the classic triumphant tales of modern medicine, told most famously in de Kruif, *Microbe Hunters*. See also Coleman, "Koch's Comma Bacillus."

34. As mentioned earlier, Koch's success enabled him to overturn the public health protocols propounded by his more socially minded predecessor, Max von Pettenkofer. But while the desire to find a coherent correlation between a pathogen and a disease entity that prompted Koch's proposal persists—as the regular appearance of new zoonotic pathogens such as HIV, SARS-CoV-I, MERS-CoV, and SARS-CoV-2 reminds us—the insufficiencies of Koch's precepts became apparent soon after they were formulated. For example, because viruses had not yet been isolated and because they cannot be grown in pure cultures, viral diseases could not be specified in Koch's terms. Furthermore, because not all organisms exposed to a particular pathogen manifest any pathology at all, the consistency of pathogen and pathology relation could not be properly predicted. Probably the most famous example of this phenomenon is Typhoid Mary, an Irish American cook who was identified as an "asymptomatic carrier" and forcibly quarantined for over twenty-five years in the first decades of the twentieth century. However, this is not merely a historical anecdote: the emergence of the new zoonotic coronavirus, SARS-Cov-2, in 2020 reminds us of this problem, since nonsymptomatic or slightly symptomatic people who harbor the virus can easily become "superspreaders." From their inception, then, Koch's postulates constituted a leaky sieve.

35. For example, molecular or evolutionary versions of the postulates have been offered. Falkow, "Molecular Koch's Postulates"; Cochran, Ewald, and Cochran, "Infectious Causation of Disease."

36. "Cholera," World Health Organization, accessed November 24, 2019, https://www.who.int/health-topics/cholera#tab=tab_1.

37. Wilcox and Colwell, "Emerging and Reemerging Infectious Diseases," 246. The authors also emphasize the importance of considering human activity: "Human activity contributed through mechanisms linked across vastly different time and space scales: human behavior and exposure to contaminated water in the household, village, or city; river basin, drainage basin, or catchment management—especially related to agriculture—affecting water quality; pathogen survival, and transport; and global climate change potentially causing more extreme weather conditions, including storm and rainfall variability in general" (248). And, of course, these are all also affected by economic, political, military, religious, and gendered variables as well.

38. Sigmund Freud articulated this insight in "On Psychical (or Mental) Treatment," his contribution to a medical handbook, *Die Gesundheit*, published in 1905:

The results of every procedure laid down by the physician and of every treatment that he undertakes are probably composed of two portions. And one of these, which is sometimes greater and sometimes less, but can never be completely disregarded, is determined by the patient's mental attitude. The faith with which he meets the immediate effect of a medical procedure depends on the one hand on the amount of his own desire to be cured, and on the other hand on his confidence that he has taken the right steps in that direction—on his general respect, that is, for medical skill—and, further, on the power which he attributes to his doctor's personality, and even on the purely human liking aroused in him by the doctor. Freud, *Standard Edition*, vol. 7, *A Case of Hysteria*, 291.

39. As mentioned earlier, Rachel Remen has contributed to this endeavor with her course the Healer's Art, now taught in scores of medical schools around the world. Narrative medicine supports and encourages physicians to recognize that the ways patients narrate the stories of their illnesses both provide crucial information about their presenting problems and offer keys to successful therapeutic interventions. Narrative medicine courses are now offered at many medical schools as well as in continuing education courses, for example, the Division of Narrative Medicine at Columbia University's Irving Medical Center (https://www.narrativemedicine.org). Rita Charon, director of Columbia's Division of Narrative Medicine, is recognized as one of the field's founding figures. Bibliographies for some of the major faculty can be found here: https://www.mhe.cuimc .columbia.edu/our-divisions/division-narrative-medicine/bibliography.

40. A number of other clinicians have also attempted to redress the reductionist orientation in medical education. One of my favorites is Cassell, *Art of Healing*.

41. While Assagioli developed his technique under the name psychosynthesis, he may not have been the first to use the term. It also appears in an important letter that Jung wrote to Freud after their famous encounter in Vienna in which Jung tried in vain to convince Freud of the reality of precognition and parapsychological phenomena: "If there is a 'psychoanalysis' there must also be a 'Psychosynthesis' which creates future events according to the same causes." McGuire, *Freud-Jung Letters*, 216. In his reply, which anticipates the break that will later come between them, Freud writes, "I also shake my wise head over Psychosynthesis and think: Yes, that's how the young people are, the only places they really enjoy visiting are those they can visit without us, to which we with our short breath and weary legs cannot follow them" (219). At this point, Assagioli and Jung were already in conversation, so it's not clear how or to whom the term first appeared.

42. Jung wrote to Freud about Assagioli in July 1909, expressing his enthusiasm for the young Italian physician: "The birds of passage are also moving in, i.e., the people who visit one. Among them is a very pleasant and perhaps valuable acquaintance, our first Italian, a Dr. Assagioli from the psychiatric clinic in Florence. Prof. Tanzi assigned him our work for a dissertation. The young man is very intelligent, seems to be extremely knowledgeable and is an enthusiastic follower, who is entering the new territory with the proper brio. He wants to visit you next spring." McGuire, *Freud-Jung Letters*, 241.

43. Freud sojourned in Paris, where he attended the lectures of the nineteenth century's most famous neurologist, Jean-Martin Charcot, precisely at the moment when Metchnikoff published his first essays on immunity as host defense. My hypothesis, for

which alas I have no proof, is that Freud's extensive use of "defense" in his psychological vocabulary derives in part from the ways Metchnikoff's innovation transformed medical thinking in the period.

44. Freud clarified this limitation very early in his career when he imagined how he would respond to a patient's objections to his technique: "'Why, you tell me yourself that my illness is probably connected with my circumstances and the events of my life. You cannot alter these in any way. How do you propose to help me, then?' And I have been able to make this reply: 'No doubt fate would find it easier than I do to relieve you of your illness. But you will be able to convince yourself that much will be gained if we succeed in transforming your hysterical misery into common unhappiness. With a mental life that has been restored to health you will be better armed against that unhappiness.'" Josef Breuer and Sigmund Freud, *Studies on Hysteria*, in Freud, *Standard Edition*, vol. 2, 305.

45. Freud, "Preface to Bourke's Scatological Rites of All Nations," in *Standard Edition*, vol. 12, *Case History of Schreber*, 337.

46. Freud, *Civilization and Its Discontents*, 11–20. Freud's critique of Rolland's sentiment, which he supposes underlies all religious sentiment, derives from his assertion: "I cannot find this 'oceanic' feeling in myself. It is not easy to deal scientifically with feelings" (12).

47. Freud, "The Question of Lay Analysis," in *Standard Edition*, vol. 20, *An Autobiographical Study*, 177–258: "The words, 'secular pastoral worker,' might well serve as a general formula for describing the function which the analyst, whether he [*sic*] is a doctor or a layman, has to perform in relation to the public" (254).

48. Blackman, *Immaterial Bodies*.

49. Theosophy is a syncretic spiritual movement founded in the late nineteenth century by Helena Blavatsky. It drew upon Neoplatonism, Hinduism, and Buddhism, which it combined with occultist tendencies within Western esoteric philosophies.

50. Assagioli, "Psychosomatic Medicine and Bio-psychosynthesis."

51. Assagioli, "Psychosynthesis." Freud used a similar analogy—albeit much more passively—in a footnote to his essay "Lines of Advance in Psycho-analytic Therapy": "After all, something similar occurs in chemical analysis. Simultaneously with the isolation of various elements induced by the chemist, syntheses which are no part of his intention come about, owing to the elective affinities of the substance concerned." Freud, *Standard Edition*, vol. 17, *Infantile Neuroses and Other Works*, 161.

52. Assagioli, *A New Method of Healing*.

53. Assagioli, *A New Method of Healing*, 6.

54. Assagioli, *A New Method of Healing*, 6.

55. Assagioli, *A New Method of Healing*, 13.

56. For a survey of these techniques, see Crampton, *Guided Imagery*; Frétigny and Virel, *L'Imagerie mentale*.

57. Freud, "Negation," in *Standard Edition*, vol. 19, *The Ego and the Id*, 235–42.

58. Assagioli, *Act of the Will*.

59. A search of Medline for "inflammatory bowel disease" and "emotion" or "affect" yielded 883,383 results. The first hit was an article in the *Journal of Crohn's and Colitis* based on a study of 201 people with Crohn's (47 percent) or other inflammatory bowel

diseases. The study concluded, "Overall the patients considered stress (84.1%), altered immunity (69.32%), family problems (49.4%), and emotional status (40.9%) as the main causes of IBD." Vengi et al., "Illness Perception."

60. Although it has had little impact on clinical practice, there actually exists a sub-subfield of biomedicine called psychoneuroimmunology that has slowly emerged over the last forty years that studies how our psyches change our biochemistry, and tries to elucidate the psychological implications of disease. It's worth thinking about the priority given to the order of syllables. How might immunoneuropsychology or immunopsycho-neurology articulate different ways of approaching mind-body function?

61. On Plato's notion that philosophy rectifies thought, see Heidegger, "On Plato's Doctrine." The Western split of body and soul arises in Plato's *Phaedo*, where it appears as a permutation of this appearance/reality opposition. If we compare ancient Greek and ancient Chinese thought systems, we find that the supposed necessity for our analytic orientation instead represents a specific cultural determination. See Jullien, "Did Philosophers Have to Become?"; Jullien, *Vital Nourishment*.

62. Isabelle Stengers argues that "interest"—which etymologically derives from *inter-esse*, being in between—articulates the field of relations that constitute "scientific practices." Practices are "scientific" insofar as they are "interesting" to those who ascribe to scientific standards. Stengers, *Invention of Modern Science*, 94–95.

63. Canguilhem, *Études d'histoire et de philosophie*, 47.

64. "Within its own limits, every discipline recognizes true and false propositions, but it repulses a whole teratology of knowledge. The exterior of a science is both more and less populated than one might think. . . . There are monsters on the prowl, however, whose forms alter with the history of knowledge." Foucault, "Discourse on Language," 223, translation corrected.

65. Moshe Feldenkrais, whose work chapter 4 engages, put the epistemic conundrum succinctly: "Is imagination a fact, a reality? Or is imagination only supposedly an imagined fact of existence?" Feldenkrais, *Elusive Obvious*, 79.

66. For an overview of the rationalism versus empiricism debates, see Markie, "Rationalism vs. Empiricism." Not coincidentally, the word *empiricism*, first used in the seventeenth century to (pejoratively) characterize medical methods based on trial and error, derives from the late Latin *empirica*, meaning remedy or medicine, which itself leaned on an earlier Greek cognate, ἐμπειρία, meaning something known from experience or by testing: *Oxford English Dictionary Online*, s.v. "empiricism, n," https://www-oed-com.proxy.libraries.rutgers.edu/view/Entry/61344?redirectedFrom=empiricism.

67. Kant, *Critique of Pure Reason*, 121–22.

68. On the history of mesmerism, see Darnton, *Mesmerism and the End*; Rausky, *Mesmer ou la révolution thérapeutic*; Roussillon, *Du baquet de Mesmer*; Chertok and Stengers, *A Critique of Psychoanalytic Reason*; Gauld, *A History of Hypnotism*, 1–38; Crabtree, *From Mesmer to Freud*. Translations of some of the documents addressed below appear in Binet and Féré, *Animal Magnetism*.

69. Stengers, "Doctor and the Charlatan," 92.

70. Ramsey, *Professional and Popular Medicine*.

71. Veaumorel, *Aphorismes de M. Mesmer*.

72. Mesmer, *Mémoire sur la découverte*, 26.

73. "Following the principles known of universal attraction, confirmed by observations which teach us that the planets mutually affect each other in their orbits, and that the moon and the sun cause and direct the flux and reflux of the sea on our globe, as well as in the atmosphere; I assert that these spheres also exercise a direct action on all the constitutive parts of animated bodies, particularly the nervous system, by means of a fluid which penetrates everything; I determined this action by the intension and remission of the properties of matter and organized bodies, such as gravity, cohesion, elasticity, irritability, and electricity.... I named the property of the animal body which renders it susceptible to the action of celestial and earthly bodies, ANIMAL MAGNETISM." Mesmer, *Mémoire sur la découverte*, 6–7.

74. On Mesmer's disputes with the Faculté concerning the appropriate manner of testing his technique, see Donaldson, "Mesmer's 1780 Proposal."

75. Hannaway, "Société Royale de Médecine and Epidemics"; Gramain-Kibleur, "Le testament de la Société Royale"; Ramsey, "Traditional Medicine and Medical Enlightenment."

76. Gramain, "Au temps de la Société Royale"; Gramain-Kibleur, "Le testament de la Société Royale."

77. Mesmer, *Précis historique des faits relatifs*, 45.

78. Mesmer expatiates upon his arguments with—and grudges against—various authorities in Austria and France in two of his publications: Mesmer, *Mémoire sur la découverte*; Mesmer, *Précis historique des faits relatifs*.

79. Golinski, "Precision Instrumentation."

80. Lavoisier, *Traité élémentaire de chimie*, ix, emphasis added. Two years prior to publishing his *Traité*, Lavoisier coauthored what may be the first chemistry textbook, *Méthod de nomenclature chimique*, which contains a very similar assertion: "the imagination . . . tends to continually lead us beyond the true.... It solicits us to draw consequences which do not derive immediately from the facts" (10–11).

81. Lavoisier, *Traité élémentaire de chimie*, x–xi.

82. Lavoisier, *Traité élémentaire de chimie*, 7.

83. Once Lavoisier's criteria proved interesting, they began to accrue interest (in both the epistemological and economic senses).

84. Mesmer, *Lettres de M. Mesmer*, 13.

85. Mesmer, *Lettres de M. Mesmer*, 14.

86. In this way, Mesmer anticipates Isabelle Stengers's perspective by two centuries: "It may be said that the 'question of the imagination' is a symptom of a practical contradiction between the constraints defining the laboratory and the modes of existence of living creatures who are interrogated there. The laboratory needs a system which will respond to a definition in terms of variables, while the beings about whom the question of the imagination is being asked 'respond' in a very different sense, according to the meaning which they themselves lend to their environment." Stengers, "Doctor and the Charlatan," 112–13.

87. Darnton, *Mesmerism and the End*, 46–126, describes the political stakes involved in the way animal magnetism circulated in France during the late eighteenth century, in-

cluding his discussion of "mesmerism as radical political theory." In the *Exposé* that Bailly read before the Académie Royale des Sciences, he articulates the political rationale: "the Sciences, which increase the truth, gain still more from the suppression of an error: an error is always a bad germ [*levain*] which ferments and corrupts the mass into which it is introduced. But when this error leaves the empire of the Sciences in order to spread over the multitude, in order to separate and agitate their minds [*esprits*], when it presents a false means of healing to the sick that prevents it from seeking other help, when above all it influences both morality and physiology, a good government is interested in destroying it." Bailly, *Exposé des expériences qui on été faites*, 4.

88. Bailly, *Rapport de commissaires chargés par le roi*; Bailly, *Rapport des commissaires de la Société Royale*.

89. Bailly, "Rapport secret sur la magnétisme animal," 92–100.

90. Bailly, *Exposé des expériences qui ont faites*.

91. Jussieu, "Rapport de l'un des commissaires."

92. Deslon produced a rebuttal to the official report: Deslon, *Observations sur les deux rapports*. In his bibliographic note, Darnton provides numerous archival sources in *Mesmerism and the End*, 171–75. For an excellent example, see the compendium of cases gathered to support animal magnetism in Eslon, *Supplément aux deux rapports*. Darnton, *Mesmerism and the End*, 3–45.

93. "These convulsions were extraordinary by their number, duration and force. As soon as one convulsion began, many others broke out. The commissioners observed these for more than three hours; they were accompanied by coughing up of cloudy and viscous fluid, torn out by the violence of their efforts. . . . These convulsions were characterized by precipitous, involuntary movements of all bodily parts and of the entire body; by contractions of the throat; by spasms of the hypochondrium and the epigastria; by the blurring and distraction of the eyes; by piercing cries, and tears, and hiccups and uncontrollable laughing. They were preceded or followed by a state of languor and dreaminess, of a kind of exhaustion and even slumber." Bailly, *Rapport des Commissaires de la Société Royale*, 6.

94. Bailly, *Rapport des commissaires de la Société Royale*, 8.

95. Bailly, *Rapport des commissaires de la Société Royale*, 11, 14.

96. Bailly, *Rapport des commissaires de la Société Royale*, 18.

97. Bailly, *Rapport des commissaires de la Société Royale*, 25.

98. Bailly, *Rapport des commissaires de la Société Royale*, 25–26, emphasis added.

99. Bailly, *Rapport des commissaires de la Société Royale*, 27.

100. Bailly, *Rapport des commissaires de la Société Royale*, 27.

101. Bailly, *Rapport des commissaires de la Société Royale*, 28.

102. Obviously, the current standard of randomized double-blind testing does not involve actual blindfolds but rather procedures designed to render both the experimenting and the experimental subjects metaphorically blind. The difficulties with these procedures are considered in the next section, on the role of the placebo in contemporary biomedicine.

103. Bailly, *Rapport des commissaires de la Société Royale*, 29–30, 31, emphasis added.

104. The report's characterization of the imagination also seems particularly indebted, as Franklin Rausky has suggested in *Mesmer ou la révolution thérapeutic*, to the great

French naturalist Georges-Louis Leclerc de Buffon's more embodied sense of imagination. This indebtedness reflects Buffon's role as the giant of eighteenth-century natural history as well as his enduring prominence within the Académie Royale des Sciences, several of whose members were among the authors of the report. It also marks the report's larger project to circumscribe the practices of legitimate—and legitimated—medicine within the domain of natural science.

Unlike the philosophical psychology of thinkers like Shaftesbury and Leibniz, who theorized the imagination as a mental faculty that considered human engagement in the world primarily as a perceptual problem (e.g., Leibniz's famous distinction in his *Nouveau Essais* [1704] between "*perceptions insensibles*" and "*la puissance active*," which founds a duality of mind), Buffon situated the imagination at and as the threshold between sensory and conceptual intelligence, thereby both recapitulating and revising the famous Cartesian duality of body and mind. Buffon introduced his discussion of the imagination in the fourth volume of his magnum opus, *Histoire Naturelle*, published in 1753. Here he applies his naturalist gaze to a comparison of humans and animals in order to "lead us to the important science of which man himself is the object." As a prelude to the section that considers human exceptionalism, under the rubric "Homo Duplex," Buffon defines the imagination as simultaneously a faculty of the soul unique to humans and as "a principle which depends only on the corporeal organs and which we have in common with animals."

105. Bailly, *Rapport des commissaires de la Société Royale*, 44, emphasis added.

106. The principle of sufficient reason, anticipated by Spinoza and first articulated by Leibniz, provides a logic that underwrites the shift from a nonmodern view that God can intervene directly in the world, for example by miracles, to one in which God governs the world through prescribed laws that are rational and hence in principle available to both description and explanation. For a summary of the principle, see Melamed and Lin, "Principle of Sufficient Reason."

107. In adhering to this assumption, the report unproblematically deploys a polemical idiom, *saine physique*—which I've translated here as "rational physics" but might more literally be rendered as "sound physics" or even "healthy physics." This idiom appeared frequently throughout the period, often in phrases—*les loix de la saine physique, les principles de la saine physique, les regles de la saine physique*—to evoke prevailing standards of rational or scientific explanation. In French, *sain* can mean sane, healthy, sound, or wholesome. When used in the phrase *saine physique*, it takes on the sense of normal, accepted, accredited, valid, or even orthodox science. However, it might also signify rational (as opposed to the irrationality of insanity), especially insofar as it works to exclude the imagination as a verifiable or even real cause. Thanks to Joan Scott for her translation help.

108. Bailly, *Rapport des commissaires*, 60.

109. These include not just bodily but also military and political effects. For example, the *Rapport des commissaires de la Société Royale* notes that the imagination comes into play in the heat of battle ("where the enthusiasm of courage as well as the terrors of panic propagate with rapidity") as well as during political upheavals ("The same cause gives birth to revolts: men united in large numbers are more susceptible to their sensations; reason

has less reign over them, and when fanaticism presides over these assemblies, it produces the Trembleurs des Cevennes"). Bailly, *Rapport des commissaires*, 53. (Trembleurs des Cevennes was a prophetic movement of Protestants during the reign of Louis XIV that arose against the persecution that followed the revocation of the Edict of Nantes in 1685.)

110. Bailly, *Rapport des commissaires de la Société Royale*, 61.

111. In French, the word *expérience* can signify both experiment and experience. This semantic play seems especially relevant in this context, since the commission's experimental setup aspired to foreclose the experiences of the experimental subjects by blinding them.

112. Motherby, *A New Medical Dictionary*.

113. Logeion, s.v. "placeo," accessed June 20, 2021, https://logeion.uchicago.edu/placeo. The history of this usage is somewhat circuitous. Derived from the future indicative of the Latin verb *placeo*, to please, to give pleasure, to be approved, to be pleasing, to be acceptable, to suit, to satisfy, *placebo* was used to translate the opening word of Psalm 116:9 (*Placebo Domino in regione vivorum*—I will please the Lord in the land of the living), which was sung in the Vespers of the medieval church's Office for the Dead and subsequently came to designate Vespers itself. This God-pleasing aspect of *placebo* was disaggregated from its ecclesiastical sense during the Middle Ages and came to mean a flatterer, sycophant, or parasite—though perhaps continuing to carry with it some trace of mortality. See *Oxford English Dictionary Online*, s.v. "placebo, n," https://www-oed-com.proxy.libraries.rutgers.edu/view/Entry/144868?redirectedFrom=placebo.

114. Shapiro and Shapiro, *Powerful Placebo*, 28–42 and 123–74.

115. Daniel Moerman proposed that the placebo effect be reconceived as a "meaning response" since, he argues, what catalyzes effects attributed to placebos are not the substances themselves but the meanings they carry. Moerman, *Meaning, Medicine and the "Placebo Effect"*; Hutchinson and Moerman, "Meaning Response, 'Placebo,' and Method."

116. Although two recent biomedical fields, psychoneuroimmunology and psychoneuroendocrinology, take this insight as their point of departure, so far they have had little impact on clinical practice. For overviews, see Ader, "Psychoneuroimmunology"; Daruna, *Introduction to Psychoneuroimmunology*. The literature on medical placebos has myriad conjectures about the specific ways that placebos induce their effects. For an overview as well as a critique, see Kaptchuk, "Open Label Placebos."

117. On the history of clinical trials, see Shapiro and Shapiro, *Powerful Placebo*, 123–74. On the placebo more generally, Guess et al., *Science of the Placebo*; Peters, *Understanding the Placebo Effect*; Brody and Brody, *Placebo Response*; Harrington, *Placebo Effect*; Shepard and Sartorius, *Non-specific Aspects of Treatment*; Spiro, *Doctors, Patients, and Placebos*; Watts, *Pleasing the Patient*; Brody, *Placebos and the Philosophy*; Jospe, *Placebo Effect in Healing*.

118. Blease and Annoni, "Overcoming Disagreement."

119. Chertok and Stengers, *A Critique of Psychoanalytic Reason*, 24.

120. Beecher, "Powerful Placebo." In 1961, a negative form of the placebo, the "nocebo," was introduced to describe the way negative expectations can deleteriously affect the outcomes of medical treatments. Kennedy, "Nocebo Reaction."

121. The literature on intentional effects of placebos as treatments, including what are being called open-label placebos, has expanded greatly in the past few years. Ted

Kaptchuk, who directs the Program in Placebo Studies, Beth Israel Deaconess Medical Center in Harvard Medical School, has been one of the main exponents of this potential. He describes how he came to conduct these studies in Kaptchuk, "Open Label Placebos." For early examples of studies, see Kaptchuk and Miller, "Placebo Effects in Medicine"; and Kaptchuk and Miller, "Open Label Placebo." Not surprising, inflammatory bowel diseases serve as key examples in these studies.

122. Over the past thirty years since Naomi introduced me to guided imagery, official medicine has expanded its limits somewhat to encompass some nonreductive modes of therapeutic intervention. A new archive suggests that there exist some practical reasons to consider that the imagination might have therapeutic resources to offer. For example, the founding of the Office of Alternative Medicine in 1992 and the subsequent establishment of the National Center for Complementary and Alternative Medicine in 1998, under the auspices of the National Institutes of Health, mark something of a sea change in official understandings about the potentials of some nondeterministic treatments. Furthermore, research articles now regularly appear in major biomedical publications on techniques like biofeedback, meditation, and acupuncture for conditions such as high blood pressure, chronic pain, migraines, incontinence, and constipation; or on the use of guided imagery for other conditions, including cancers, asthma, arthritis, coronary disease, diabetes, fibromyalgia, headache, and inflammatory bowel disease; along with considerations of such practices as journal keeping and creative writing as therapeutic modalities. (Not surprisingly, much of the interest in these techniques appears in the highly gendered domain of nursing, along with the slightly less gendered domains of psychotherapy and psychiatry.) Alas, this recognition of the imagination only obtains insofar as such practical knowledge doesn't trouble the epistemological premises on which official medicine depends.

123. Nevertheless, appealing to medical legitimacy today, just as when Mesmer did so more than two hundred years ago, requires conforming to the standards of evaluation that medicine deems rational, even though these might not exhaust the possibilities for considering how we can support the healing process. For example, when acupuncturists first attempted to demonstrate that their methods could provide demonstrable therapeutic results, and hence that they should be eligible for insurance reimbursements, they were forced to introduce control techniques (for example, creating sham needles that stuck to but didn't really penetrate the skin) in order to conform to the standards of blind testing. Unfortunately, these couldn't be randomly controlled double-blind tests because those providing the treatments always knew the difference. Furthermore, the criteria acupuncturists used to evaluate outcomes were different from those used by biomedical experts.

124. Foucault, *Society Must Be Defended*, 9.

## CHAPTER FOUR. WHEN WE LEARN TO HEAL, IT MATTERS

1. The first official use of *AIDS* occurred in *Morbidity and Mortality Weekly Report* in 1982 (CDC, "Current Trends Update").

2. In my senior year in high school, out of nine hundred students I was voted both biggest brain and biggest mouth—the only person to get two body parts—so clearly I had a soft spot for the head.

3. Descartes, *Meditations on First Philosophy*.

4. Although I didn't know this at the time, Descartes, who also wrote *The Passions of the Soul*, had a more complex understanding of the human organism, especially in relation to questions of health and illness, with which he was somewhat obsessed. See Shapin, "Descartes the Doctor."

5. Reese, *Moshe Feldenkrais*. All biographical information about Feldenkrais comes from this monumental work by one of Feldenkrais's students.

6. Feldenkrais, *Potent Self*, 81.

7. "The brain is capable of a greater variety of patterns of situations than we actively employ; only those patterns become operative that personal experience of the self and the world have facilitated and made recurrent or potentially available." Feldenkrais, *Potent Self*, 127. In a way, this represents part of Feldenkrais's rejoinder to Freud. Whereas Freud noticed that hysterical paralysis conformed to the ideation of bodily movement, rather than to its physiology, Feldenkrais noticed that habitual movement often entailed internal conflicts that were not just physiological but ideational. For Feldenkrais, ideation, like all movement, is embodied.

8. Feldenkrais makes this clear in his discussion of posture in *The Potent Self*: "We will always have to allow for the fact that every act has not only (1) the normal physiological and mechanical difficulties to be overcome through learning, but also (2) the ever-present adult whose approval must be sought and met. All these normal conditions make it practically impossible to learn anything without linking it to an affect, a sort of third eye, which watches our mobilization of means and reinstates the original corrective influence in most details. The result is that we screw ourselves up to do things and thus come to associate with all action a sensation of effort. The internal resistance then becomes part and parcel of the action, and a necessary component to perform it" (58).

9. Feldenkrais, *Potent Self*, 92. Feldenkrais's observation resonates with Freud's similar conclusions in *Civilization and Its Discontents*, although he foregrounds physiology rather than psychology. Needless to say, the two do not remain distinct for either Freud or Feldenkrais.

10. Mauss, in "Les techniques des corps," includes the cultural variations in modes of walking as part of his "biographical enumeration of bodily techniques" (14).

11. Feldenkrais, *Potent Self*: "One walks in a particularly inappropriate manner for reasons dictated by a distorted dependence relationship to other people" (124).

12. Feldenkrais, *Potent Self*, 126.

13. To my mind toilet training, which Feldenkrais occasionally mentions (e.g., *Potent Self*, 86), provides an even better example of the complex physio-psychosocial patternings that shape infant development—and that groove in a lifetime of psycho-neuromuscular propensities—in a context of absolute biological, economic, and emotional dependence. Gilles Deleuze and Félix Guattari refer to these kinds of physio-psychosocial patternings as "coding the flows" (*Anti-Oedipus*, 141). "The social machine is literally a machine, irrespective of any metaphor, inasmuch as it exhibits an immobile motor, and undertakes a variety of interventions: flows are set apart, elements are detached from a chain, and portions of the tasks to be performed are distributed. Coding the flows implies all these operations."

14. Feldenkrais was deeply influenced by the work of Émile Coué, a French pharmacist and psychologist who developed a technique of "autosuggestion" in the early twentieth century that anticipated Assagioli's use of guided imagery. In his work as a pharmacist, Coué observed that his enthusiastic recommendations often enhanced the efficacy of the prescriptions he administered, a sort of placebo effect *avant la lettre*. He also studied hypnosis with Hippolyte Bernheim, with whom Freud also studied and whose book on hypnotic suggestion Freud translated with commentary. Through his engagement with Coué, Feldenkrais began to appreciate the capacity for the imagination to help us augment and enhance our physical capacities. His first publication was a translation of an English book about Coué (Harry C. Brooks's *The Practice of Autosuggestion*), to which Feldenkrais appended two chapters of his own. Feldenkrais, *Thinking and Doing*.

In the course of his scientific work, Feldenkrais befriended a number of well-known Marxists, including crystallographer J. D. Bernal, zoologist Solly Zuckerman, and physicist Frédéric Joliot-Curie. While never identifying as such himself, Feldenkrais opened his first book, *Body and Mature Behavior* (1949), with a Left critique of Freud that concludes, "It is hard to deny that the traditional foundations of our social structure need thorough revision. No objective observer, free of prejudice, will argue against the necessity of radical changes. . . . In such changes lie hope for a better future" (10).

15. Feldenkrais, *Potent Self*, 155.

16. Feldenkrais, *Elusive Obvious*, 70.

17. Feldenkrais, *Potent Self*, 238.

18. Feldenkrais, *Elusive Obvious*, 79–80.

19. "One has to set about learning to learn as is befitting for the most important business in human life." Feldenkrais, *Potent Self*, xxxix.

20. "The therapeutic value of any method can be gauged by just this—the contribution it makes to the learning of the function in which the person is impotent." Feldenkrais, *Potent Self*, xli.

21. Feldenkrais, *Potent Self*, 110–11. Feldenkrais coins "cerebrosomatic" in *Potent Self*, 53.

22. Gordon, "Tenacious Assumptions in Western Medicine," 19–56.

23. Feldenkrais, *Potent Self*, 67.

24. Feldenkrais, *Potent Self*, 127.

25. Feldenkrais, *Potent Self*, 11.

26. Feldenkrais, *Embodied Wisdom*, 88.

27. Feldenkrais, *Elusive Obvious*, 117. Feldenkrais remained skeptical of curing, holding that "cure" does not constitute an appropriate healing objective because "to be cured means to return to [a] past mode of functioning, but life is a process, and an irreversible process at that." Feldenkrais, *Body Awareness as Healing Therapy*, 37.

28. "My contention is that learning always involves the whole frame, and all learning that does not directly involve muscular activity is poor. . . . The basis of all learning is the reciprocity between mind and body, which is the conventional way of expressing the fact that the nervous system and the body are one whole organism. The experience of the body is necessary to form the linking of the nervous mechanisms with reality." Feldenkrais, *Elusive Obvious*, 130–31.

29. This is precisely Feldenkrais's critique of the fallacy embedded in the idea of cure: "Cure is a return to a previously enjoyed state of activity which need not have been excellent or even good. The habitual and the familiar we do not question; improvement we grade. The former is the automatic background of your system; the latter is the foreground of our awareness. The two are different dimensions. One is an atavistic sensation; the other is learned knowledge that gives us freedom of choice—which is the major prerogative of Homo Sapiens." Feldenkrais, *Body Awareness as Healing Therapy*, 37.

30. Feldenkrais's ethos rhymes for me with Foucault's emphasis on forms of subjectification. Subjectification for Foucault does not only entail a cognitive dimension but always situates living human beings in relation to themselves and others. Indeed, his critique of Althusser's notion of ideology—despite Althusser's insistence on its "materiality"—stems precisely from its abstract orientation. Foucault undertakes his critique of ideology throughout his books and lectures beginning in the mid-1970s. *Discipline and Punish* and *The History of Sexuality*, vol. 1, provide good examples of Foucault's position.

31. On the fallacy of importing individualism's political significance into biology, see Margulis and Sagan, *Slanted Truths*.

32. Gordon, "Tenacious Assumptions in Western Medicine," 19–56.

33. In *Discipline and Punish*, Foucault details the profusion of disciplinary techniques developed in the eighteenth and nineteenth centuries that "links the singular and the multiple. It allows the characterization of the individual as individual and the ordering of a given multiplicity" (135–69, 149).

34. For introductions to the concept of qi, see Hall and Ames, "Qi"; Chen, "Qi (C'hi)." See also Rošker, "Concept of *Qi*."

35. In *Body and Mature Behavior*, Feldenkrais alludes to this possibility but doesn't pursue it: "The whole problem is a social one and reeducation has much better prospects of success if conducted in groups and not in the seclusion and pretended secrecy of the consulting room" (218).

36. Wavy Gravy, né Hugh Nanton Romney Jr., is a peace activist, organizer, and entertainer whose life trajectory cut across many of the milestones of the 1960s counterculture. For a quick summary of his many adventures, see his Wikipedia page, accessed July 20, 2020; https://en.wikipedia.org/wiki/Wavy_Gravy#Camp_Winnarainbow. For the history of the property, see the Camp Winnarainbow website, accessed July 20, 2020; https://www.campwinnarainbow.org/about-us/our-story/.

37. In 1984, California Proposition 41 was overwhelmingly defeated, 63 percent to 37 percent. "California Proposition 41, Limits on Welfare Spending (1984)," Ballotpedia, accessed July 19, 2021, https://ballotpedia.org/California_Proposition_41,_Limits_on _Welfare_Spending_(1984).

38. Piero Ferrucci has become a renowned international teacher of psychosynthesis. See Ferrucci, *What We May Be*; Ferrucci, *Inevitable Grace*; Ferrucci, *Beauty and the Soul*; Ferrucci, *Your Inner Will*.

39. For an excellent introduction to Emilie Conrad and her work, check out her memoir, *Life on Land* (2007).

40. Dennis Stock, Unknown title, photograph, 1955, Pinterest, https://www.pinterest .com/pin/218917231860193274/.

41. After her death, Continuum, like many other somatics programs led by charismatic teachers (including Feldenkrais and Rolfing) split into competing factions. The current practice that legally owns the name "Continuum Movement" does not represent the ethos I describe here. Instead, the spirit of Continuum as I know it has been carried on by Susan Harper (see Continuum Montage, https://www.continuummontage.com), who was Emilie's coteacher and business partner for several decades, as well as a number of other longtime Continuum teachers (see Continuum Teachers Directory, https://www.continuumteachers.com/teachers).

42. The next section explains why this might be the case; however, an example that suggests this concept is feminist consciousness raising (CR). In the 1960s and '70s, as women came together to share their experiences of female socialization in CR groups, they created value contexts in which what they had heretofore taken as individual frustration, limitation, or oppression could now be recognized as the systematic effects of sexism. This revaluation of individual experience as an effect of collective devaluation made it possible for women to transform their conditions individually and collectively. Indeed, one consequence of this transvaluation of values—to invoke Nietzsche—was to reveal that the notion of the individual itself represented a cultural value that fails to appreciate the complex situation within which women's oppression comes to seem so natural. As a practice dating from the same period and primarily taught by women to other women—and not too many of us men—Continuum partakes of a similar CR ethos.

43. In many ways, Emilie's insights about movement echoed those of Henri Bergson (discussed in chapter 1). Like Bergson, Emilie believed "the living being is above all a thoroughfare, and . . . the essence of life is in the movement by which life is transmitted." Or, as Emilie often put it, in what I came to think of as the Continuum bumper sticker: "Movement is not what we do, movement is what we are." While I know Emilie had read Bergson, I don't know how much she was inspired by him in framing her practice. However, it seems more than just random coincidence that she gave the name Continuum to her work, given that Bergson held, "If we suppose an extended *continuum*, and in this *continuum*, the center of real action, which is represented by our body, its activity will appear to illuminate all those parts of matter with which at each successive moment it can deal." Bergson, *Matter and Memory*, 232–33.

44. Mind-body is the idiom of Candace Pert, the neuroscientist who discovered opiate receptors. Pert, *Molecules of Emotion*.

45. One of Emilie's touchstone texts was Norman O. Brown's *Love's Body*.

46. For an excellent introduction to Susan Harper and her work, check out this hour-long documentary: Elaine Colandrea, *Heart of Continuum*," Vimeo, 2020, video, 1:03:05, https://vimeo.com/449520710.

47. Marcuse, *Eros and Civilization*. "The performance principle, which is that of an acquisitive and antagonistic society in the process of constant expansion, presupposes a long development during which domination has been increasingly rationalized: control over social labor now reproduces society on a large scale and under improving conditions. . . . Men do not live their own lives but perform pre-established functions. While they work, they do not fulfill their own needs and faculties but work in *alienation*" (45).

48. "Possessive individualism" is the idiom introduced by Canadian political theorist C. B. Macpherson. See Macpherson, *Political Theory of Possessive Individualism*.

49. Feldenkrais, *Embodied Wisdom*, 42.

50. Michel Foucault describes this discipline process as the production of "docile bodies." Foucault, *Discipline and Punish*, 135–94.

51. Simondon uses the idiom "internal resonance" to evoke the harmonization of disparate systems (physical, vital, psychic, and social) in the process of individuation: "Internal resonance is the most primitive mode of communication between realities of different orders; it contains a double process of amplification and condensation." Simondon, *L'individuation psychic et collective*, 67.

52. Heidegger, "Onto-theo-logical Constitution of Metaphysics," 42–74.

53. *Metaphysics* literally means "beyond *phusis* [φύσις]," originally referring to the works in Aristotle's corpus arranged after his writings about the natural world. In Homeric Greek, *phusis* initially referred to the growth of plants—like *viriditas*—which then came to refer more widely to "nature" in opposition to *nomos* (νόμος) as the human-oriented sphere of custom and law. Logeion, s.v. "φύσις," accessed August 8, 2020, https://logeion.uchicago.edu/φύσις; Logeion, s.v. "νόμος," accessed August 8, 2020, https://logeion.uchicago.edu/νόμος.

54. In their book *What Is Philosophy?*, Gilles Deleuze and Félix Guattari offer a succinct definition of philosophy: "knowledge through pure concepts" (7).

55. Some four hundred years after Plato, his body/soul dichotomy provided Christianity with a schema for Platonizing Judaism, which then heralded Christianity's "good news," proclaiming that the soul's "eternal life" persists after the body's death. While the split of body and soul characterizes Western ontotheology, it does not exist in all systems of thought. In his brilliant book *Vital Nourishment*, François Jullien juxtaposes Western and Chinese thinking to demonstrate the cultural limitations of this seemingly self-evident Western binary.

56. Hylomorphism derives from the etymons *hule* (ὕλη), which in ancient Greek means "wood" and by metonymy "matter or material," and *morphé* (μορφή), form or shape. Logeion, s.v. "ὕλη," accessed August 8, 2020, https://logeion.uchicago.edu/ὕλη; Logeion, s.v. "μορφή," accessed August 8, 2020, https://logeion.uchicago.edu/μορφή.

57. Van der Eijk, "Aristotle's Psycho-physiological Account."

58. Simondon, *L'individu et sa genèse physico-biologique*; Simondon, *L'individuation psychic et collective*. For a captivating extrapolation from and development of this critique, see Steigler, *Technics and Time, 1*.

59. Simondon, *L'individuation psychic et collective*, 16.

60. Simondon, *L'individuation psychic et collective*, 13. Bovier and den Hollander, *Metastability*.

61. Simondon, *L'individuation psychic et collective*, 13.

62. Simondon, *L'individuation psychic et collective*, 12.

63. The physicist Erwin Schrödinger defined living systems as those that homeostatically maintain negative entropy. Schrödinger, *What Is Life?*

64. Simondon, *L'individuation psychic et collective*, 12.

65. Simondon, *L'individuation psychic et collective*, 17.

66. Simondon, *L'individuation psychic et collective*, 18–19.

67. "Psychic being cannot resolve its own [vital] problematic within itself. Its charge of preindividual reality, at the same time that it individuates as a psychic individual which exceeds the living individual and incorporates the living into a system of world and the subject, permits participation in the form of a condition of collective individuation. Individuation in the form of the collective makes the individual a group individual, associated with a group by virtue of the preindividual reality that it carries within it and which, joined with that of other individuals, *individuates itself in a collective unity*. These two individuations, psychic and collective, are reciprocal, one in relation to the other; they allow us to define the category of the transindividual which can be used to account for the systematic unity of interior individuation (psychic) and exterior individuation (collective). The psycho-social world of the transindividual is neither social fact nor inter-individual; it supposes a real operation of individuation departing from a preindividual reality, associated with individuals and capable of constituting a new problematic with its own metastability." Simondon, *L'individuation psychic et collective*, 19–20.

68. This interpretation of Simondon is indebted to that of Bernard Stiegler, who in many works underscores the relation between "subsistence," "existence," and "consistence," holding that "the transindividual opens existence to planes of consistence." Stiegler, *What Makes Life Worth Living?*, 67. See, for example, the section titled "Subsistence, Existence and Consistence" in Stiegler, *Disbelief and Discredit*, 1:89–93.

69. "The psyche is composed of successive individuations that permit the being to resolve problematic states corresponding to the establishment of permanent connections between what is larger and smaller than itself. But the psyche cannot resolve these itself at the level of the individual alone; it is the basis of a participation in a much greater individuation, that of the collective. Putting itself into question, the individual being cannot go beyond the limits of anxiety, an operation without action, a permanent emotion which never resolves affectivity, an experience through which the individuated being explores the limits of its being without the power to go beyond them. *The notion of the transindividual corresponds to the collective taken as an axiomatic resolving the psychic problematic.*" Simondon, *L'individuation psychic et collective*, 22.

70. Freud, *Civilization and Its Discontents*. Following Bernard, Koch, and Pasteur, who represented the cutting edge of medical science at the time of his medical training and his work in a neurology lab, Freud believed that the individual is the sine qua non of civilization. The original German word *Kultur* translated as "civilization" in the book's English title refers more specifically to the self-improving activities (*Bildung*) undertaken by individuals of the German middle classes. On the distinction between civilization and culture in the context of French aristocratic (*civilité*) and German bourgeois (*Kultur*) circles, see Elias, *Civilizing Process: Sociogenetic and Psychogenetic Investigations*.

71. Freud, "Three Essays on the Theory of Sexuality," in *Standard Edition*, vol. 7, *A Case of Hysteria*, 162.

72. Josef Breuer and Sigmund Freud, *Studies on Hysteria*, in Freud, *Standard Edition*, vol. 2, 305.

73. Gilles Deleuze refers to this kind of immaterial causality as "quasi-cause." Riffe, "Deleuze's Concept of Quasi-cause," 278–94.

74. On the importance of breathing to a nonreductive philosophy, see the essays collected in Škof and Berndtson, *Atmospheres of Breathing*.

75. On the historical evolution of the idea that the body contains the self, see Elias, *Civilizing Process: History of Manners*. Elias posed the question of "self-containment" as follows: "Is the body the vessel which holds the true self locked within it? Is the skin the frontier between inside and outside? What in man is the capsule, and what the encapsulated?" (282).

76. Obviously, *spirit* has a plethora of meanings. The *Oxford English Dictionary* underscores this plethora when it tells us that *spirit* derives from the "classical Latin *spiritus*, action of breathing, respiration, breath, (final) breath; (in grammar) aspiration, air, life, consciousness, soul, vital principle animating the world, divine inspiration, essential quality, nature, disposition, ardent disposition, enthusiasm, vigor, arrogance, pride, wind, breeze, wind in the stomach or bowels, scent, perfume, odor; in post-classical Latin also the Holy Spirit, evil spirit, demon (Vetus Latina), soul of a dead person, ghost, angel, incorporeal or immaterial being, courage, tendency, inclination, emotional part of a person," and so on.

Given this range of possible significance, spirituality seemed a tad too promiscuous to me, covering a multitude of sins without ever getting to the heart of the matter.

77. Simondon, *L'individuation psychic et collective*, 101. In his final volume of lectures at the Collège de France, Michel Foucault also takes up the problem of the "other life" (*autre vie*) and the "true life" by juxtaposing the philosophical attitudes of Plato's Socrates to those of Diogenes the Cynic. Foucault, *Courage of the Truth*.

78. Simondon, *L'individuation psychic et collective*, 105.

79. Simondon, *L'individuation psychic et collective*, 105. In the final lines of the final volume of his lectures at the Collège de France, Michel Foucault made a similar gesture toward articulating the "other" life within the "same": "But what I would like to stress in conclusion is this: there is no establishment of the truth without an essential position of otherness; the truth is never the same; there can be truth only in the form of the other world and the other life [*l'autre monde et de la vie autre*]." Foucault, *Courage of the Truth*, 340. Foucault's own discussion of spirituality as a transformative truth practice—which he distinguished from philosophy—appears in Foucault, *Hermeneutics of the Subject*, 16–17.

80. François Jullien argues that Western philosophy's investment in construing the world in terms of mutually exclusive oppositions betrays a cultural bias not familiar to ancient Chinese thinking, characterized by the complementarity of contraries. Jullien, "Did Philosophers Have to Become Fixated?"

81. On the potential for community rather than immunity, see my essays "A Cure for COVID-19," and "COVID and the Death Drive"; Cohen, Boler, and Davis, "The Biopolitics of Pandemics"; and my earlier article "Immune Communities, Common Immunities."

82. Winnicott, *Playing and Reality*. Winnicott develops the notions of transitional objects and transitional phenomena as key elements of his theories of child development, known generally as object relations. Winnicott extrapolated these ideas to his notion of play, which he identifies as one of the most important elements of both developmental

and therapeutic relationships. Winnicott's critical insight about transitional phenomena is that they conform neither to the logic of identity nor to the logic of noncontradiction. Hence, they partake of what Simondon called the "preindividual." In transitional phenomena, self and other, inside and outside, subjective and objective, do not oppose one another, but rather "interweave," thereby opening up creative possibilities that play realizes: "This gives us our indication for therapeutic procedure—to afford possibility for formless experience, and for creative impulses, motor and sensory, which are the stuff of playing. And on the basis of playing is built our whole experiential existence. No longer are we either introvert or extrovert. We experience life in the area of transitional phenomena, in the exciting interweave of subjectivity and objective observation, and in an area that is intermediate between the inner reality of the individual and the shared reality of the world that is external to individuals" (86).

Play serves as the prevailing impulse during the all-nighter precisely because it braids the individual with the collective and thus precipitates a spiritual mode of transindividuation (which, as Simondon argues, affirms "the meaning of being as separate and connected, as alone and as a member of the collective; the individuated being is simultaneously on its own and not on its own").

83. Logeion, s.v. "sacer," accessed August 26, 2020, https://logeion.uchicago.edu/sacer. In *The Courage of the Truth*, his final series of lectures at the Collège de France, given shortly before he died of AIDS in 1984, Foucault traces the dynamic between "this life" and "the other life" and considers the philosophical possibility that the other life might arise within this life to the thinking of Socrates and Diogenes the Cynic.

84. "In playing, and perhaps only in playing, the child or adult is free to be creative." Winnicott, *Playing and Reality*, 53.

85. Jonathan Crary argues that the continuous temporalities of digital capitalism disrupt our capacities to dream, whereas during an all-nighter dreaming together—whether we are asleep or awake—is of the essence. Crary, *24/7*.

86. Obviously, many spiritual practices from diverse cultures and traditions cultivate group meditation, breathing, chanting, prostrations, and other sacred movements. They also ritually frame the shared spaces and times in which they practice, designating these collective processes as transitional ones—whether in Winnicott's sense or not. The efficacy of all such spiritual technologies might lie in something like their ability to create, in Simondon's terms, a collective internal resonance. If so, they function as modes of transindividuation by constituting participants as "group individuals" whose physical, vital, psychic, and social individuations increasingly coincide—if not harmonize—as they participate in shared somatic practices. For, as Simondon puts it, "the collective will individuate itself in reconnecting the separated being," and that is, after all, what makes a collective a collective and not just a series of separate individuals. In the case of all-nighters, we introduce conditions that explicitly seek to disrupt the habituated haptic dimensions of individualism by playing with other modes of physical, vital, psychic, and social attunement. The practice invokes nonfamiliar ways of going-on-being-together in order to evoke vital capacities that routinely appear—or disappear—as without value or interest.

87. Edelstein and Edelstein, *Asclepius* remains the classic text on Asclepius, along with Kerényi, *Asklepios*. Since these books appeared, the scholarly literature on Asclepius and

Asclepian healing has exploded. For more recent examples, see, among others, Hart, *Asclepius*; Wickkiser, *Asklepios, Medicine*; Petsalis-Diomidis, *Truly beyond Wonders*; Renberg, *Where Dreams May Come*; Steger, Saar, and Verlag, *Asclepius*; Ploeg, *Impact of the Roman Empire*.

88. Petridou, "Asclepius the Divine Healer." On the Christian war on paganism, see Nixey, *Darkening Age*.

89. Risse, "Asclepius at Epidaurus"; Alexia Petsalis-Diomidis, in *Truly beyond Wonders*, provides much more detailed accounts of what she calls the ritual "choreography."

90. Ahearne-Kroll, "Afterlife of a Dream." Ahearne-Kroll's essay provides a wonderful explication of the temple practice of dream healing, from the ritual approach to its precincts through the process of dream incubation to the dream decoding by the temple priests and its subsequent renarrativization as a carved inscription that can then endure for hundreds if not thousands of years beyond the dream as its "afterlife."

91. Edelstein and Edelstein, *Asclepius*, 65; O'Donnell, *Pagans*.

92. Staden, "Jesus and Asklepios."

93. Foucault, *Society Must Be Defended*, 7–9.

94. Traditional histories of medicine often contrasted Hippocratic and Asclepian therapies as if the former anticipated modern rational medicine while the latter represented an atavistic attachment to the irrational. More recently, scholars of antiquity have troubled this sharp distinction by noticing the ways in which the practices not only coexisted for over a millennium but also mutually recognized each other's specificity. Jouanna, "Hippocrates and the Sacred"; van der Eijk, "'Theology' of the Hippocratic Treatise"; Lloyd, *Magic, Reason, and Experience*; Edelstein and Edelstein, *Asclepius*, 139–41.

95. However, it also represents an archival problem: ancient practitioners in the Hippocratic tradition elaborated a doctrine about which they wrote voluminously, and many of these texts have been preserved as part of the Hippocratic corpus. Asclepian temple healing, on the other hand, produced no doctrines or texts, and most of what we know about it depends on interpreting archaeological artifacts, including the stone stelae which record testimonials to the cures that Asclepius effected. However, the lack of textual documentation alone does not explain why Asclepian practices no longer feature in our thinking about how to heal.

96. Edelstein and Edelstein, *Asclepius*, 125.

97. Morris, "Un-forgetting Asclepius," 426.

98. The Edelsteins underscore Benveniste's etymological argument: "The ancients understood the role of the physician not only as that of a personal advisor and helper. They believed that the doctor in taking care of the patient assumed the responsibility which the superior has for his subordinates, the king for his subjects; he was supposed to act as the guardian of the patient who gave himself over into the tutelage of the doctor." Edelstein and Edelstein, *Asclepius*, 111–12.

99. Jouanna, *Hippocrates*, 181. "The Hippocratic physicians allied themselves with the enlightened minds of the Periclean age who promoted the new rationalism and criticized—sometimes strenuously—those who believed that a disease could be caused by the intervention of a particular divinity, contrasting the notion of divine causality to rational causality. The rational attitude of these physicians is all the more remarkable since

belief in the efficacy of magical practices and in the gods as healing agents is well attested in the popular mentality of the age, at the height of the fifth century."

100. Typically, *phusis* is opposed to *nomos*, meaning custom or law. Thus, the claim that physicians derived their knowledge from nature is a "customary" claim if there ever was one.

101. Of course, this putative alliance with nature rather than gods never held entirely true, since Greek medicine often continued to affirm the divinity of all nature. Yet because physicians invested in the possibility of knowing the causes of diseases, nature's divinity must conform to structures of human knowledge. Hankison, "Magic, Religion, and Science."

102. Vernant, *Myth and Thought*; Vernant and Vidal-Naquet, *Myth and Tragedy*; Vernant, *Myth and Society*; Jouanna, "Le médicin modèle du législateur"; Jouanna, "Médicine et politique."

103. Detienne, *Masters of Truth*, 12, 136.

104. Kerényi, *Asklepios*, 34.

105. Kerényi, *Asklepios*, 34.

106. Not coincidentally, Asclepius the god of healing incorporates these same contraries in his mythic origins. While a number of ancient texts, beginning with the *Iliad*, mention Asclepius as a healing figure, his classic mythography appears in Pindar's third *Pythian Ode*. According to Pindar, Asclepius was the son of Apollo and a mortal princess, Coronis, who while pregnant with Apollo's child became infatuated with a fellow mortal, Ischys. Unfortunately for her, jealous Apollo had her under surveillance and, discovering her betrayal, sent his sister Artemis to kill Coronis—which she did, slaughtering Coronis along with her neighbors. However, in the aftermath, Apollo suffered (some) remorse, and when her family placed her body upon the funeral pyre, he dived into the flames, and "in one step he reached the child and snatched it from the corpse; the burning fire divided its blaze for him, and he bore the child away and gave him to the Magnesian Centaur to teach him to heal many painful diseases for men." Chiron the Centaur (half human, half horse) was a renowned healer who also tutored Achilles and taught Asclepius his arts so that Asclepius became capable of "tending some of them with gentle incantations, others with soothing potions, or by wrapping remedies all around their limbs, and others he set right with surgery." Alas, Asclepius was not immune to greed and, being paid to raise a man from the dead, he so incensed Zeus that Zeus killed him with a lightning bolt. In Pindar, then, Asclepius appears as a trickster figure whose existence blurs the same boundaries that Greek philosophy and Greek medicine were in the process of determining as fixed oppositions: child of god and mortal, born from death, tutored by a man/horse, killed by Zeus when he raised the dead, only to return to the living as a god who could restore the dying to life, Asclepius incorporates the persistence of the ambiguities that medical rationality has always sought to purify. Given his backstory, it makes sense that the epiphanic Asclepian cure reminds the petitioner that healing naturally manifests the divine, or at least the unknown, if not the unknowable. Pindar, *Odes*, edited by Diane Arnson Svarlien, 1990, Perseus Digital Library, accessed September 1, 2020, http://www.perseus.tufts.edu/hopper/text?doc =Perseus%3Atext%3A1999.01.0162%3Abook%3DP.%3Apoem%3D3. Other versions of

the mythography also appear in Hygenus Astronomus, *Astronomica* 2.14.1.1, PHI *Latin Texts*, accessed September 6, 2020, https://latin.packhum.org/loc/899/1/0#23; Apollodorus, *The Library 3*, translated by J. G. Frazer, *Theoi*, accessed September 1, 2020, https://www.theoi.com/Text/Apollodorus3.html#10; and Ovid, *Metamorphoses*; among others.

107. Cohen, "Self, Not-Self."

CODA. HEALING WITH COVID, OR WHY MEDICINE IS NOT ENOUGH

1. Pope Francis, "A Crisis Reveals What Is in Our Hearts," *New York Times*, November 26, 2020, https://www.nytimes.com/2020/11/26/opinion/pope-francis-covid.html.

# Bibliography

Abram, David. "The Mechanical and the Organic: On the Impact of Metaphor in Science." In *Scientists on Gaia*, edited by Stephen H. Schneider and Penelope J. Boston, 66–74. Cambridge, MA: MIT Press, 1991.

Ader, Robert. "Psychoneuroimmunology." In *International Encyclopedia of the Social and Behavioral Sciences*, edited by Neal Smelser and Paul Baltes, 12422–48. Oxford: Pergamon, 2001.

Ahearne-Kroll, Stephen P. "The Afterlife of a Dream and the Ritual System of the Epidaurian Asklepieion." *Archiv für Religionsgeschichte* 15, no. 1 (2014): 35–52.

Asad, Talal. "Thinking about the Secular Body, Pain, and Liberal Politics." In *Living and Dying in the Contemporary World*, edited by Clara Han and Veena Das, 337–53. Oakland: University of California Press, 2016.

Assagioli, Roberto. *The Act of the Will*. New York: Viking, 1973.

Assagioli, Roberto. *A New Method of Healing: Psychosynthesis*. New York: Lucis, 1927.

Assagioli, Roberto. "Psychosomatic Medicine and Bio-psychosynthesis." Lecture given at International Psychosomatic Week, Rome, 1967. Available at Synthesis Center, https://www.synthesiscenter.org/articles/0121.pdf.

Assagioli, Roberto. "Psychosynthesis: Individual and Social (Some Suggested Lines of Research)." Association for the Advancement of Psychosynthesis, 2017. https://www.aap-Psychosynthesis.org/resources/Documents/individual_and_social.pdf.

Atlan, Henri. "Knowledge of Ignorance." In *Forms of Living: On Self-Organization, Philosophy, Bioethics and Judaism*, edited by Stefanos Geroulanos and Todd Meyers, 384–89. New York: Fordham University Press, 2011.

Bailly, Jean Sylvain. *Exposé des expériences qui ont faites pour l'examen du magnétisme animal*. Paris: Imprimerie-Librarie de la Reine et de l'Académie Royale des Sciences, 1784.

Bailly, Jean Sylvain. *Rapport des commissaires chargés par le roi, de l'examen du magnétisme animal*. Paris: Imprimerie Royale, 1784.

Bailly, Jean Sylvain. *Rapport des commissaires de la Société Royale de Médecine, nommé par le roi, pour faire l'examen du magnétisme animal*. Paris: Imprimerie-Librarie de la Reine, et de l'Académie Royale des Sciences, 1784.

Bailly, Jean Sylvain. "Rapport secret sur la magnétisme animal, redigé par Bailly au nom de la meme commission." In *Histoire académique du magnétisme animal*, edited by Charles Burdin and Frédéric Dubois, 91–101. Paris: Ballière, 1841.

Bazerman, Charles. *Shaping Written Knowledge: Genre and Activity of the Experimental Article in Science*. Madison: University of Wisconsin Press, 1980.

Beecher, Henry K. "The Powerful Placebo." *Journal of the American Medical Association* 159, no. 17 (1955): 1602–6.

Behr, Marcel A., Maziar Divangahi, and Jean-Daniel Lalande. "What's in a Name? The (Mis)Labelling of Crohn's as an Autoimmune Disease." *Lancet* 376 (2010): 202–3.

Benveniste, Émile. "La doctrine médicale des Indo-Européens." *Revue de l'histoire des religions* 130 (1945): 5–12.

Bergson, Henri. *Creative Evolution*. Translated by Arthur Mitchell. New York: Modern Library, 1944 [1907].

Bergson, Henri. *The Creative Mind*. Translated by Mabelle Andison. Westport, CT: Greenwood, 1946.

Bergson, Henri. *Matter and Memory*. Translated by Nancy Margaret Paul and W. Scott Palmer. New York: Zone, 1991.

Bernard, Claude. *Introduction à l'étude de la médicine expérimentale*. Edited by François Dagognet. Paris: Garnier-Flammarion, 1966 [1865].

Bernard, Claude. *Principes de médecine expérimentale*. Edited by Léon Delhoume. Paris: Presses Universitaires de France, 1947.

Bichat, Marie-François-Xavier. *Recherches physiologiques sur la vie et la mort*. Paris: Charpentier, 1852.

Binet, Alfred, and Charles Féré. *Animal Magnetism*. New York: D. Appleton, 1888.

Blackman, Lisa. *Immaterial Bodies: Affect, Embodiment, Mediation*. Los Angles: Sage, 2012.

Blease, Charlotte, and Marco Annoni. "Overcoming Disagreement: A Roadmap for Placebo Studies." *Biology and Philosophy* 34, no. 18 (2019).

Bovier, Anton, and Frank den Hollander. *Metastability: A Potential-Theoretic Approach*. New York: Springer, 2015.

Breslaw, Elaine. *Lotions, Potions, Pills and Magic: Health Care in Early America*. New York: NYU Press, 2012.

Brier, Jennifer. *Infectious Ideas: U.S. Political Responses to the AIDS Crisis*. Chapel Hill: University of North Carolina Press, 2009.

Brisou, Bernard. "Saigon, Nha-Trang, Hanoi: Le service de santé colonial et les débuts des Instituts Pasteur d'Indochine." *Revue Historique des Armées* 208, no. 3 (1997): 17–28.

Brody, Howard. *Placebos and the Philosophy of Medicine: Clinical, Conceptual and Ethical Issues*. Chicago: University of Chicago Press, 1980.

Brody, Howard, and Daralyn Brody. *The Placebo Response: How You Can Release the Body's Inner Pharmacy for Better Health*. New York: Cliff Street, 2000.

Brooks, Harry C. *The Practice of Autosuggestion by the Method of Emile Coué*. Translated by Moshe Feldenkrais. New York: Dodd, Mead, 1922.

Brown, Norman O. *Love's Body*. New York: Random House, 1966.

Buffon, Georges Leclerc de. *Histoire naturelle, générale et particulière.* 15 vols. Paris: Imprimerie Royal, 1749–1767.

Burnet, Frank MacFarlane. *The Clonal Selection Theory of Acquired Immunity.* London: Cambridge University Press, 1959.

Burnet, Frank Macfarlane. *Self and Not-Self: Cellular Immunology, Book One.* London: Cambridge University Press, 1969.

Canguilhem, Georges. *Études d'histoire et de philosophie des sciences concernant les vivants et la vie.* Paris: Vrin, 1994.

Canguilhem, Georges. "Health: Crude Concept and Philosophical Question." *Public Culture* 20, no. 3 (2008): 467–77.

Canguilhem, Georges. "The Idea of Nature in Medical Theory and Practice." In *Writings on Medicine*, translated by Stefanos Geroulanos and Todd Meyers, 25–33. New York: Fordham University Press, 2012.

Canguilhem, Georges. *Knowledge of Life.* Translated by Stefanos Geroulanos and Daniela Ginsberg. New York: Fordham University Press, 2008.

Canguilhem, Georges. *The Normal and the Pathological.* Translated by Carolyn Fawcett. New York: Zone, 1985.

Canguilhem, Georges. "Une pédagogie de guérison, est-elle possible?" *Nouvelle revue de psychoanalyse*, no. 17 (1978): 13–26.

Canon, Walter. "Physiological Regulation of Normal States: Some Tentative Postulates Concerning Biological Homeostatics." In *À Charles Richet: Ses amis, ses collègues, ses élèves*, edited by Auguste Pettit, 91–93. Paris: Les Éditions Médicales, 1926.

Carel, Havi. *Illness: The Cry of the Flesh.* London: Routledge, 2013.

Cassell, Eric. *The Art of Healing.* New York: Oxford University Press, 2013.

CDC. "A Cluster of Kaposi's Sarcoma and Pneumocystis carinii Pneumonia among Homosexual Male Residents of Los Angeles and Orange Counties, California." *Morbidity and Mortality Weekly Report* 31, no. 23 (June 18, 1982): 305–7. https://www.cdc.gov/mmwr/preview/mmwrhtml/00001114.htm.

CDC. "Current Trends Update on Acquired Immune Deficiency Syndrome (AIDS)—United States." *Morbidity and Mortality Weekly Report* 31, no. 37 (September 24, 1982): 507–8, 513–14. https://www.cdc.gov/mmwr/preview/mmwrhtml/00001163.htm.

Chamberlin, William, and Saleh Naser. "Integrating Theories of the Etiology of Crohn's Disease: On the Etiology of Crohn's Disease: Questioning the Hypotheses." *Medical Science Monitor* 12, no. 2 (2006): 27–33.

Chen, Chung-Ying. "Qi (C'hi)." In *Encyclopedia of Chinese Philosophy*, edited by Antonio Cua, 615–17. New York: Routledge, 1993.

Chertok, Léon, and Isabelle Stengers. *A Critique of Psychoanalytic Reason: Hypnosis as a Scientific Problem from Lavoisier to Lacan.* Translated by Martha Noel Evans. Stanford, CA: Stanford University Press, 1992.

Clarke, Adele, Janet K. Shim, Laura Mamo, Jennifer Ruth Fosket, and Jennifer R. Fishman. "Biomedicalization: Technoscientific Transformations of Health, Illness, and U.S. Biomedicine." *American Sociological Review* 68, no. 2 (2003): 161–94.

Clavreul, Jean. *L'ordre médical.* Paris: Éditions du Seuil, 1978.

Cochran, Gregory M., Paul W. Ewald, and Kyle D. Cochran. "Infectious Causation of Disease: An Evolutionary Perspective." *Perspectives in Biology and Medicine* 43, no. 3 (2000): 406–48.

Cohen, Ed. *A Body Worth Defending: Immunity, Biopolitics and the Apotheosis of the Modern Body*. Durham, NC: Duke University Press, 2009.

Cohen, Ed. "Covid and the Death Drive of Toxic Individualism." In *Pandemic Exposures: Economy and Society in the Time of Corona Virus*, edited by Didier Fassin and Marion Fourcade, 433–46. Chicago: Hau Books, 2021.

Cohen, Ed. "A Cure for Covid-19 Will Take More Than Personal Immunity." *Scientific American*, August 7, 2020. https://www.scientificamerican.com/article/a-cure-for-covid-19-will-take-more-than-personal-immunity/.

Cohen, Ed. "Immune Communities, Common Immunities." *Social Text* 26, no. 1 (2008): 95–114.

Cohen, Ed. "Live Thinking, or the Psychagogy of Michel Foucault." *differences* 25, no. 2 (2004): 1–32.

Cohen, Ed. "Self, Not-Self, but Not Not-Self: The Knotty Paradoxes of Autoimmunity: A Genealogical Rumination." *Parallax* 23, no. 1 (2017): 28–45.

Cohen, Ed, Megan Boler, and Elizabeth Davis. "The Biopolitics of Pandemics: Interview with Ed Cohen." *Cultural Studies* 36, no. 3 (2022): 396–409.

Coleman, William. "Koch's Comma Bacillus: The First Year." *Bulletin of the History of Medicine* 6, no. 3 (1987): 315–42.

Conrad, Emilie. *Life on Land: The Story of Continuum, the World-Renowned Self-Discovery and Movement Method*. Berkeley, CA: North Atlantic Books, 2007.

Cosnes, Jacques, Corinne Gower-Rousseau, Philippe Seksik, and Antoine Cortot. "Epidemiology and Natural History of Inflammatory Bowel Diseases." *Gastroenterology* 140, no. 6 (2011): 1785–94.

Crabtree, Adam. *From Mesmer to Freud: Magnetic Sleep and the Roots of Psychological Healing*. New Haven, CT: Yale University Press, 1993.

Crampton, Martha. *Guided Imagery: A Psychosynthesis Approach*. Montreal: Quebec Center for Psychosynthesis, 1974.

Crary, Jonathan. *24/7: Late Capitalism and the Ends of Sleep*. New York: Verso, 2014.

Craver, Carl, and James Tabery. "Mechanisms in Science." In *The Stanford Encyclopedia of Philosophy*, edited by Edward N. Zalta. Spring 2017. https://plato.stanford.edu/archives/spr2017/entries/science-mechanisms/.

Crohn, Burrill B., Leon Ginzburg, and Gordon Oppenheimer. "Regional Ileitis: A Pathologic and Clinical Entity." *Journal of the American Medical Association* 99, no. 16 (1932): 1323–29.

Crohn, Burrill B., and Henry Janowitz. "Reflections on Regional Ileitis, Twenty Years Later." *Journal of the American Medical Association* 156, no. 13 (1954): 1221–25.

Darnton, Robert. *Mesmerism and the End of the Enlightenment in France*. Cambridge, MA: Harvard University Press, 1968.

Daruna, Jorge H. *Introduction to Psychoneuroimmunology*. 2nd ed. Amsterdam: Elsevier Academic Press, 2012.

de Kruif, Paul. *Microbe Hunters*. New York: Blue Ribbon, 1926.

Deleuze, Gilles, and Félix Guattari. *Anti-Oedipus: Capitalism and Schizophrenia.* Translated by Robert Hurley, Mark Seem, and Helen Lane. Minneapolis: University of Minnesota Press, 1983.

Deleuze, Gilles, and Félix Guattari. *What Is Philosophy?* Translated by Hugh Tomlinson and Graham Burchill. London: Verso, 1994.

Deny, Keith. "Evidence-Based Medicine and Medical Authority." *Journal of Medical Humanities* 20, no. 4 (1999): 247–63.

Derkatch, Colleen. "Method as Argument: Boundary Work in Evidence-Based Medicine." *Social Epistemology* 22, no. 4 (2008): 371–88.

Derrida, Jacques. *Life Death.* Translated by Pascale-Anne Brault and Michael Naas. Chicago: University of Chicago Press, 2020.

Derrida, Jacques. "Plato's Pharmacy." In *Dissemination,* translated by Barbara Johnson, 61–171. Chicago: University of Chicago Press, 1981.

Descartes, René. *Meditations on First Philosophy, with Selections from the Objections and Replies.* Translated by John Cottingham. Cambridge: Cambridge University Press, 1996.

Deslon, Charles. *Observations sur les deux rapports de MM. les commissaires nommés par sa majesté, pour l'examen du magnétisme animal par M. Deslon.* Paris: Chez Clousier, 1784.

Deslon, C. N. *Supplément aux deux rapports de MM. les commissaires de l'Académie et de la Faculté de Médecine, et de la Société Royal de Médecine.* Amsterdam: n.p., 1785.

Detienne, Marcel. *The Masters of Truth in Archaic Greece.* Translated by Janet Lloyd. New York: Zone, 1996.

Dijck, José van. *Transparent Body: A Cultural Analysis of Medical Imaging.* Seattle: University of Washington Press, 2005.

Donaldson, I. M. L. "Mesmer's 1780 Proposal for a Controlled Trial to Test His Method of Treatment Using 'Animal Magnetism.'" *Journal of the Royal Society of Medicine* 98, no. 12 (2005): 572–75.

Dosse, François. *Gilles Deleuze and Félix Guattari: Intersecting Lives.* Translated by Deborah Glassman. New York: Columbia University Press, 2010.

Dossey, Larry. *Space, Time, and Medicine.* Boston: New Science Library, 1985.

Dumit, Joseph. *Drugs for Life: How Pharmaceutical Companies Define Our Health.* Durham, NC: Duke University Press, 2012.

Edelstein, Emma J., and Ludwig Edelstein. *Asclepius: Collection and Interpretation of the Testimonies.* Vols. 1 and 2. Baltimore: Johns Hopkins University Press, 1998.

Ehrenreich, Barbara, and Dierdre English. *Witches, Midwives, and Nurses: A History of Women Healers.* 2nd ed. New York: Feminist Press, 2010.

Ehrlich, Paul. *Studies in Immunity.* Translated by Charles Bolduan. New York: John Wiley, 1910.

Elias, Norbert. *The Civilizing Process.* Vol. 1, *The History of Manners.* Translated by Edmund Jephcott. New York: Pantheon, 1982.

Elias, Norbert. *The Civilizing Process: Sociogenetic and Psychogenetic Investigations.* Translated by Edmund Jephcott. London: Blackwell, 2000.

Enders, Giulia. *Gut: The Inside Story of Our Body's Most Underrated Organ.* New York: Greystone, 2018.

Engel, George L. "The Need for a New Medical Model: A Challenge for Biomedicine." *Science* 196, no. 4286 (1977): 129–38.

Epstein, Steven. *Impure Science: AIDS, Activism, and the Politics of Knowledge.* Berkeley: University of California Press, 1996.

Falkow, Stanley. "Molecular Koch's Postulates Applied to Microbial Pathogenicity." *Reviews of Infectious Diseases* 10, no. S2 (1988): S274–76.

Farley, John. "Parasites and the Germ Theory of Disease." *Millbank Quarterly* 67, suppl. 1 (1989): 50–68.

Farman, Abou. *On Not Dying: Secular Immortality in the Age of Technoscience.* Minneapolis: University of Minnesota Press, 2020.

Fawcett, Jacqueline. "Thoughts about Meanings of Compliance, Adherence, and Concordance." *Nursing Science Quarterly* 33, no. 4 (2020): 358–60.

Feldenkrais, Moshe. *Body and Mature Behavior: A Study of Anxiety, Sex, Gravitation, and Learning.* Berkeley, CA: Frog, 2005.

Feldenkrais, Moshe. *Body Awareness as Healing Therapy: The Case of Nora.* Berkeley, CA: North Atlantic, 1993.

Feldenkrais, Moshe. *The Elusive Obvious: The Convergence of Movement, Neuroplasticity, and Health.* Berkeley, CA: North Atlantic, 2019.

Feldenkrais, Moshe. *Embodied Wisdom: The Collected Papers of Moshe Feldenkrais.* Edited by Elizabeth Beringer. Berkeley, CA: North Atlantic, 2010.

Feldenkrais, Moshe. *The Potent Self: A Study of Spontaneity and Compulsion.* Berkeley, CA: Frog, 1985.

Feldenkrais, Moshe. *Thinking and Doing: A Monograph by Moshe Feldenkrais.* Longmont, CO: Genesis II, 2013.

Ferrucci, Piero. *Beauty and the Soul: The Extraordinary Power of Everyday Beauty to Heal Your Life.* New York: TarcherPerigee, 2010.

Ferrucci, Piero. *Inevitable Grace: Breakthroughs in the Lives of Great Men and Women: Guides to Your Self-Realization.* New York: TarcherPerigee, 2009.

Ferrucci, Piero. *What We May Be: Techniques for Psychological and Spiritual Growth through Psychosynthesis.* New York: TarcherPerigee, 2009.

Ferrucci, Piero. *Your Inner Will: Finding Personal Strength in Critical Times.* New York: TarcherPerigee, 2015.

Fett, Sharla. *Working Cures: Healing, Health and Power on Southern Slave Plantations.* Chapel Hill: University of North Carolina Press, 2002.

Fiocchi, Claudio. "Inflammatory Bowel Disease Pathogenesis: Where Are We?" *Journal of Gastroenterology and Hepatology* 30, suppl. 1 (2015): 12–18.

Flexner, Abraham. *The American College: A Criticism.* New York: Century, 1908.

Flexner, Abraham. *Medical Education in the United States and Canada: A Report to the Carnegie Foundation for the Advancement of Teaching.* Bulletin no. 4. New York: Carnegie Foundation for the Advancement of Teaching, 1910.

Folwaczny, Christian, Jurgen Glas, and Helga-Paula Torok. "Crohn's Disease: An Immunodeficiency?" *European Journal of Gastroenterology and Hepatology* 15, no. 6 (2003): 621–26.

Foucault, Michel. *The Birth of the Clinic: An Archaeology of the Medical Perception.* Translated by A. M. Sheridan Smith. New York: Vintage, 1994.

Foucault, Michel. *The Courage of the Truth: The Government of Self and Others II. Lectures at the Collège de France, 1983–1984*. Translated by Graham Burchell. New York: Palgrave, 2011.

Foucault, Michel. *Discipline and Punish: The Birth of the Prison*. Translated by Alan Sheridan. New York: Vintage, 1977.

Foucault, Michel. "Discourse on Language." In *The Archaeology of Knowledge and The Discourse on Language*. Translated by A. M. Sheridan Smith, 215–37. New York: Pantheon, 1972.

Foucault, Michel. *The Hermeneutics of the Subject: Lectures at the Collège de France, 1981–1982*. Translated by Graham Burchell. New York: Palgrave Macmillan, 2005.

Foucault, Michel. *The History of Sexuality*. Vol. 1, *An Introduction*. Translated by Robert Hurley. New York: Vintage, 1990.

Foucault, Michel. "Impossible Prison." Translated by Colin Gordon. In *Foucault Live: Collected Interviews, 1961–1984*, edited by Sylvère Lotringer, 275–86. New York: Semiotext(e), 1996.

Foucault, Michel. *Les machines à guérir: Aux origines de l'hôpital modern*. Paris: Pierre Margada, 1979.

Foucault, Michel. "Polemics, Politics, and Problematizations." In *The Essential Works of Foucault, 1954–1984*. Vol. 1, *Subjectivity and Truth*. Edited by Paul Rabinow, 111–20. New York: New Press, 1997.

Foucault, Michel. *The Politics of Truth*. Translated by Lisa Hochroth and Catherine Porter. Los Angeles: Semiotext(e), 2007.

Foucault, Michel. "Preface to the History of Sexuality, vol. 2." In *The Foucault Reader*, edited by Paul Rabinow. New York: Pantheon, 1984.

Foucault, Michel. *Society Must Be Defended: Lectures at the College de France, 1975–1976*. Translated by David Macey. New York: Picador, 1997.

Foucault, Michel. "The Subject and Power." *Critical Inquiry* 8, no. 4 (1982): 777–95.

Foucault, Michel. "Truth and Juridical Forms." In *Power: Essential Works of Foucault, 1954–1984*. Translated by Robert Hurley. New York: New Press, 2000.

Foucault, Michel. "Truth, Power and Self: An Interview." In *Technologies of the Self*, edited by Luther Martin, Hugh Gutman, and Patrick Hutton. Amherst: University of Massachusetts Press, 1988.

Fowler, James, ed. *A Dictionary of Practical Medicine*. Philadelphia: P. Blakiston, 1890.

Frank, Arthur W. *At the Will of the Body: Reflections on Illness*. Boston: Houghton Mifflin, 1991.

Frétigny, Roger, and André Virel. *L'Imagerie mentale: Introduction à l'onirotherapie*. Geneva: Éditions du Mont Blanc, 1968.

Freud, Sigmund. *Civilization and Its Discontents*. Translated by James Strachey. New York: Norton, 1961.

Freud, Sigmund. *The Standard Edition of the Complete Psychological Works of Sigmund Freud*. Edited and translated by James Strachey. London: Hogarth, 1953–1974.

Fride, Ester. "The Endocannabinoid-CB(1) Receptor System in Pre- and Postnatal Life." *European Journal of Pharmacology* 500, no. 1–3 (2004): 289–97.

Furness, J. B. *The Enteric Nervous System*. Oxford: Wiley-Blackwell, 2006.

Gaitán, Adriana V., JodiAnne T. Wood, Fan Zhang, Alexandros Makriyannis, and Carol J. Lammi-Keefe. "Endocannabinoid Metabolome Characterization of Transitional and Mature Human Milk." *Nutrients* 10, no. 9 (2018): 1294.

Gaudillière, Jean-Paul. *Inventer la biomédecine: La France, l'Amerique et la productions des savoirs du vivant*. Paris: Éditions la Découverte, 2002.

Gauld, Alan. *A History of Hypnotism*. London: Cambridge University Press, 1992.

Geison, Gerald. *The Private Science of Louis Pasteur*. Princeton, NJ: Princeton University Press, 1995.

Gieryn, Thomas F. "Boundary-Work and the Demarcation of Science from Non-science: Strains and Interests in Professional Ideologies of Scientists." *American Sociological Review* 48, no. 6 (1983): 781–95.

Gieryn, Thomas F. *Cultural Boundaries of Science: Credibility on the Line*. Chicago: University of Chicago Press, 1999.

Glocker, Erik, and Bodo Grimbacher. "Inflammatory Bowel Disease: Is It a Primary Immunodeficiency?" *Cellular and Molecular Life Sciences* 69 (2012): 41–48.

Golinski, Jan. "Precision Instrumentation and the Demonstrative Order of Proof in Lavoisier's Chemistry." *Osiris* 9, no. 1 (1994): 30–47.

Gordon, Deborah. "Tenacious Assumptions in Western Medicine." In *Biomedicine Examined*, edited by Margret Lock and Deborah Gordon, 19–56. Dordrecht: Kluwer Academic, 1988.

Gramain, Pascale. "Au temps de la Société Royale de Médecine." *Médecine/Sciences* 29 (2013): 656–63.

Gramain-Kibleur, Pascale. "Le testament de la Société Royale de Médecine." *Revue général de droit médical* 9 (2003): 63–82.

Greco, Monica. "On Illness and Value: Biopolitics, Psychosomatics, Participating Bodies." *Medical Humanities* 45, no. 2 (2019): 107–15.

Greco, Monica. "On the Art of Life: A Vitalist Reading of Medical Humanities." In *Un/knowing Bodies*, edited by Joanna Latimer and Michael Schillmeier, 25–45. London: Wiley-Blackwell, 2009.

Greco, Monica. "Vitalism Now—A Problematic." *Theory, Culture, and Society* 38, no. 2 (2021): 47–69.

Groddeck, Georg. *The Book of the It*. 1923. Reprint, New York: International Universities Press, 1976.

Guénel, Annick. "The Creation of the First Overseas Pasteur Institute." *Medical History* 43, no. 1 (1999): 1–25.

Guess, Harry A., Linda Engel, Arthur Kleinman, and John Kusek, eds. *Science of the Placebo: Toward an Interdisciplinary Research Agenda*. London: BMJ, 2002.

Hacking, Ian. *Historical Ontology*. Cambridge, MA: Harvard University Press, 2002.

Hacking, Ian. *The Taming of Chance*. Cambridge: Cambridge University Press, 1990.

Hall, David L., and Roger T. Ames. "Qi." In *Routledge Encyclopedia of Philosophy*, edited by Edward Craig, 862–63. New York: Routledge, 1998.

Han, Clara, and Veena Das. "Introduction: A Concept Note." In *Living and Dying in the Contemporary World*, edited by Clara Han and Veena Das, 1–37. Oakland: University of California Press, 2016.

Hankinson, R. J. "Magic, Religion, and Science: Divine and Human in the Hippocratic Corpus." *Apeiron* 31, no. 1 (1998): 1–34.

Hannaway, Caroline. "The Société Royale de Médecine and Epidemics in the Ancien Régime." *Bulletin of the Society of Medicine* 46, no. 3 (1972): 257–73.

Haraway, Donna J. "The Biopolitics of Postmodern Bodies." In *Cyborgs, Simians and Women*, 203–30. New York: Routledge, 1991.

Harrington, Anne, ed. *The Placebo Effect: An Interdisciplinary Approach*. Cambridge, MA: Harvard University Press, 1997.

Hart, Gerald D. *Asclepius: The God of Medicine*. London: Royal Society of Medicine, 2000.

Haynes, R. Brian, and David L. Sackett, eds. *Compliance with Therapeutic Regimes*. Baltimore: Johns Hopkins University Press, 1976.

Heidegger, Martin. "On Plato's Doctrine of the Truth." In *Pathmarks*, edited by William McNeill, 155–82. New York: Cambridge University Press, 1998.

Heidegger, Martin. "The Onto-theo-logical Constitution of Metaphysics." In *Identity and Difference*, translated by Joan Stambaugh, 42–74. New York: Harper and Row, 1969.

Hoefer, Carl. "Causal Determinism." In *The Stanford Encyclopedia of Philosophy*, edited by Edward N. Zalta. Spring 2016. http://plato.stanford.edu/archives/spr2016/entries/determinism-causal/.

Hutchinson, Phil, and Daniel Moerman. "The Meaning Response, 'Placebo,' and Method." *Perspectives in Biology and Medicine* 61, no. 3 (2018): 361–78.

Jerne, Niels K. "The Immune System." *Scientific American* 229, no. 1 (1973): 52–63.

Jones, Howel L., and J. E. Lennard-Jones. "Corticosteroids and Corticotropin in the Treatment of Crohn's Disease." *Gut* 7, no. 2 (1966): 181–87.

Jones, W. H. S. *Hippocrates II*. Loeb Classical Library. Cambridge, MA: Harvard University Press, 1923.

Jospe, Michael. *The Placebo Effect in Healing*. Lexington, MA: Lexington, 1978.

Jouanna, Jacques. *Hippocrates*. Translated by M. B. DeBevoise. Baltimore: Johns Hopkins University Press, 1999.

Jouanna, Jacques. "Hippocrates and the Sacred." In *Greek Medicine from Hippocrates to Galen: Selected Papers*, edited by Philip van der Eijk, translated by Neil Allies, 97–118. Leiden: Brill, 2012.

Jouanna, Jacques. "Médecine et politique dans la *Politique* d'Aristote." *Ktèma* 5 (1980): 257–66.

Jouanna, Jacques. "Le médecin modèle du législateur dans les *Lois*." *Ktèma* 3 (1978): 77–91.

Jullien, François. "Did Philosophers Have to Become Fixated on Truth?" Translated by Janet Lloyd. *Critical Inquiry* 28, no. 4 (2002): 803–24.

Jullien, François. *Vital Nourishment: Departing from Happiness*. Translated by Arthur Goldhammer. New York: Zone, 2007.

Jussieu, M. de. "Rapport de l'un des commissaires chargés par le roi, de l'examen du magnétisme animal." In *Histoire académique du magnétisme animal*, edited by Charles Burdin and Frédéric Dubois, 146–88. Paris: Ballière, 1841.

Kane, Race. *Pleasure Consuming Medicine: The Queer Politics of Drugs*. Durham, NC: Duke University Press, 2009.

Kant, Immanuel. *Critique of Pure Reason*. Translated by J. M. D. Meiklejohn. Electronic Classics Series. Hazleton, PA: Penn State University, 2010.

Kaptchuk, Ted. "Open Label Placebos: Reflections on a Research Agenda." *Perspectives on Biology and Medicine* 61, no. 3 (2018): 311–34.

Kaptchuk, Ted J., and Franklin G. Miller. "Open Label Placebo: Can Honestly Prescribed Placebos Evoke Meaningful Therapeutic Benefits?" *British Medical Journal* 363 (2018): k3889.

Kaptchuk, Ted J., and Franklin G. Miller. "Placebo Effects in Medicine." *New England Journal of Medicine* 373, no. 1 (2015): 8–9.

Kay, Lily E. *Who Wrote the Book of Life?: A History of the Genetic Code*. Stanford, CA: Stanford University Press, 2000.

Kennedy, W. P. "The Nocebo Reaction." *Medical World* 95 (September 1961): 203–5.

Kenny, Eimear E., Itsik Peer', Amir Karban, Laurie Ozelius, Adele A. Mitchell, Sok Meng Ng, Monica Erazo, et al. "A Genome-Wide Scan of Ashkenazi Jewish Crohn's Disease Suggests Novel Susceptibility Loci." *PLoS Genetics* 8, no. 3 (2012).

Kerényi, Károly. *Asklepios: Archetypal Image of the Physician's Existence*. Translated by Ralph Manheim. New York: Pantheon, 1959.

Kevles, Bettyann Holtzmann. *Naked to the Bone: Medical Imaging in the Twentieth Century*. New Brunswick, NJ: Rutgers University Press, 1997.

Kleinman, Arthur. *The Illness Narratives: Suffering, Healing, and the Human Condition*. New York: Basic, 1988.

Koch, Robert. "The Etiology of Anthrax, Founded on the Course of Development of the Bacillus Anthracis" (1876). In *Essays of Robert Koch*, edited and translated by K. Codell Carter, 1–17. New York: Greenwood, 1987.

Kyriakidis, Nikolaos C., Andrés López-Cortés, Eduardo V. González, Alejandra Barreto Grimaldos, and Esteban Ortiz Prado. "SARS-CoV-2 Vaccines Strategies: A Comprehensive Review of Phase 3 Candidates." *NPJ Vaccines* 6, no. 28 (2021).

Lacan, Jaques. *Les quatre concepts fondamenteaux de la psychoanalyse: Seminar XI*. Paris: Éditions du Seuil, 1973.

Latour, Bruno. *The Pasteurization of France*. Translated by Alan Sheridan and John Law. Cambridge, MA: Harvard University Press, 1988.

Latour, Bruno, and Vincent Antonin Lépinay. *The Science of Passionate Interests: An Introduction to Gabriel Tarde's Economic Anthropology*. Chicago: Prickly Paradigm, 2009.

Lavoisier, Antoine. *Méthod de nomenclature chimique*. Paris: Chez Cuchet, 1787.

Lavoisier, Antoine. *Traité élémentaire de chimie*. Vol. 1. Paris: Chez Cuchet, 1789.

Lloyd, Geoffrey Ernest Richard. *Magic, Reason, and Experience: Studies in the Origins and Development of Greek Science*. Cambridge: Cambridge University Press, 1979.

Macpherson, C. B. *The Political Theory of Possessive Individualism: From Hobbes to Locke*. Oxford: Clarendon, 1962.

Marcuse, Herbert. *Eros and Civilization: A Philosophical Inquiry into Freud*. Boston: Beacon, 1955.

Marder, Michael. "On the Vegetal Verge (with Saint Hildegard)." *Comparative and Continental Philosophy* 11, no. 2 (2019): 137–46.

Margulis, Lynn, and Dorion Sagan. *Slanted Truths: Essays on Gaia, Symbiosis, and Evolution.* New York: Springer-Verlag, 1997.

Markie, Peter. "Rationalism vs. Empiricism." In *The Stanford Encyclopedia of Philosophy*, edited by Edward N. Zalta. Fall 2017. https://plato.stanford.edu/archives/fall2017/entries/rationalism-empiricism/.

Matzinger, Polly. "The Evolution of the Danger Theory." *Expert Reviews in Clinical Immunology* 8, no. 4 (2012): 311–17.

Matzinger, Polly. "Friendly and Dangerous Signals: Is the Tissue in Control?" *Nature Immunology* 8, no. 1 (2007): 10–13.

Mauss, Marcel. "Les techniques des corps." *Journal de Psychologie Normale et Pathologique* 32, no. 3–4 (1934): 1–34.

Mayer, Emeran A. "Gut Feelings: The Emerging Biology of Gut-Brain Communication." *Nature Reviews: Neuroscience* 12, no. 8 (2011): 453–66.

Mazumdar, Pauline. *Species and Specificity: An Interpretation of the History of Immunology.* New York: Cambridge University Press, 1995.

McDermott, Michael F., and Ivona Aksentijevich. "The Autoinflammatory Syndromes." *Current Opinion in Allergy and Clinical Immunology* 2 no. 6 (2002): 511–16.

McGuire, William, ed. *The Freud-Jung Letters: The Correspondence between Sigmund Freud and Carl Jung.* Princeton, NJ: Princeton University Press, 1974.

Melamed, Yitzhak Y., and Martin Lin. "Principle of Sufficient Reason." In *The Stanford Encyclopedia of Philosophy*, edited by Edward N. Zalta. Summer 2021. https://plato.stanford.edu/archives/sum2021/entries/sufficient-reason/.

Meloni, Maurizio. "Plasticity before Plasticity: The Humoralist Body." In *Impressionable Biologies: From the Archaeology of Plasticity to the Sociology of Epigenetics*, 35–66. New York: Routledge, 2019.

Mesmer, Franz Anton. *Lettres de M. Mesmer à M. Vicq-d'Azyr et à Messieurs les auteurs du Journal de Paris.* Brussels: n.p., 1784.

Mesmer, Franz Anton. *Mémoire sur la découverte du magnétisme animal.* Geneva: Didot le Jeune, 1779.

Mesmer, Franz Anton. *Précis historique des faits relatifs au magnétisme animal.* London: n.p., 1781.

Metchnikoff, Élie. "Yeast Disease of Daphnia." In *Three Centuries of Microbiology*, edited by Hubert A. Lechevalier and Morris Solotorovsky, 188–95. New York: Dover, 1974.

Meyers, Greg. *Writing Biology.* Madison: University of Wisconsin Press, 1990.

Moerman, Daniel. *Meaning, Medicine and the "Placebo Effect."* Cambridge: Cambridge University Press, 2002.

Molodecky, Natalie A., Ing Shian Soon, Doreen M. Rabi, William A. Ghali, Mollie Ferris, Greg Chernoff, Eric I. Benchimol, et al. "Increasing Incidence and Prevalence of the Inflammatory Bowel Diseases with Time, Based on Systematic Review." *Gastroenterology* 142, no. 1 (2012): 46–54.

Morris, David B. "Un-forgetting Asclepius: An Erotics of Illness." *New Literary History* 38, no. 3 (2007): 419–41.

Motherby, G. *A New Medical Dictionary, or a General Repository of Physic.* 2nd ed. London: J. Johnson, 1785.

Moulin, Anne Marie. "Patriarchal Science: The Network of the Overseas Pasteur Institutes." In *Science and Empires: Historical Studies about Scientific Development and European Expansion,* edited by Patrick Petitjean, Catherine Jami, and Anne-Marie Moulin, 307–22. Dordrecht: Kluwer Academic, 1992.

Nagel, Thomas. *The View from Nowhere.* New York: Oxford University Press, 1986.

Nahin, Richard, Patricia Barnes, and Barbara Stussman. "Expenditures on Complementary Health Approaches: United States, 2012." *National Health Statistics Reports* 95 (2016): 1–11.

Neuburger, Max. *The Doctrine of the Healing Power of Nature throughout the Course of Time.* Translated by Linn John Boyd. New York: American Institute of Homeopathy, 1932.

Nietzsche, Friedrich. *On the Genealogy of Morality.* Translated by Carol Diethe. Cambridge: Cambridge University Press, 2007 [1887].

Nietzsche, Friedrich. "On Truth and Non-truth in an Extra Moral Sense." In *On Truth and Untruth and Other Selected Writings,* translated by Taylor Carmen, 15–50. New York: Harper Perennial, 2010.

Nietzsche, Friedrich. *The Will to Power.* Translated by Walter Kaufmann and R. J. Hollingdale. New York: Vintage, 1968.

Nixey, Catherine. *The Darkening Age: The Christian Destruction of the Classical World.* Boston: Houghton Mifflin Harcourt, 2017.

Normandin, Sebastian, and Charles T. Wolfe, eds. *Vitalism and the Scientific Image in Post-Enlightenment Life Science, 1800–2010.* Dordrecht: Springer Netherlands, 2013.

O'Donnell, James J. *Pagans: The End of Traditional Religion and the Rise of Christianity.* New York: HarperCollins, 2015.

O'Rourke, Meghan. *The Invisible Kingdom: Reimagining Chronic Illness.* New York: Riverhead, 2022.

Orrego, Fernando, and Carlos Quintana. "Darwin's Illness: A Final Diagnosis." *Notes and Records of the Royal Society* 61, no. 1 (2007): 23–29.

Ovid. *Metamorphoses.* Translated by Rolfe Humphries. Bloomington: Indian University Press, 2018.

Øyri, Styrk Furnes, Györgyi Műzes, and Ferenc Sipos. "Dysbiotic Gut Microbiome: A Key Element of Crohn's Disease." *Comparative Immunology, Microbiology and Infectious Diseases* 43 (2015): 36–49.

Pasteur, Louis. "Sur les maladies virulentes, et en particuliaer sur la maladie appelée vulgairement choléra des poules." In *Oeuvres,* vol. 6, 291–312. Paris: Masson, 1933.

Pastorelli, Luca, Carlo De Salvo, Joseph R. Mercado, Maurizio Vecchi, and Theresa T. Pizarro. "Central Role of the Gut Epithelial Barrier in the Pathogenesis of Chronic Intestinal Inflammation." *Frontiers in Immunology* 4, no. 280 (2013).

Patton, Cindy. *Sex and Germs: The Politics of AIDS.* Boston: South End, 1985.

Paulley, J. W. "The Death of Albert Prince Consort: The Case against Typhoid Fever." *QJM* 86, no. 12 (1993): 837–41.

Pelis, Kim. "Prophet for Profit in French North Africa: Charles Nicolle and the Pasteur Institute of Tunis, 1903–1936." *Bulletin of the History of Medicine* 71, no. 4 (1997): 583–622.

Pert, Candace. *Molecules of Emotion: The Science behind Mind-Body Medicine.* New York: Scribner, 1997.

Peters, David, ed. *Understanding the Placebo Effect in Complementary Medicine: Theory, Practice, and Research.* New York: Churchill Livingstone, 2001.

Petridou, Georgia. "Asclepius the Divine Healer, Asclepius the Divine Physician: Epiphanies as Diagnostic and Therapeutic Tools." In *Medicine and Healing in the Ancient Mediterranean World,* edited by Demetrios Michaelides, 291–301. Oxford: Oxbow, 2014.

Petryna, Adriana. *When Experiments Travel: Clinical Trials and the Global Search for Human Subjects.* Princeton, NJ: Princeton University Press, 2009.

Petsalis-Diomidis, Alexia. *Truly beyond Wonders: Aelius Aristides and the Cult of Asklepios.* Oxford: Oxford University Press, 2010.

Phillips, Adam. *On Kissing, Tickling and Being Bored: Psychoanalytic Essays on the Unexamined Life.* Cambridge, MA: Harvard University Press, 1993.

Plevy, Scott, and Stephen Targan. "Future Therapeutic Approaches for Inflammatory Bowel Diseases." *Gastroenterology* 140, no. 6 (2011): 1838–46.

Ploeg, Ghislaine E. van der. *The Impact of the Roman Empire on the Cult of Asclepius.* Leiden: Koninklijke Brill, 2018.

Ramsey, Matthew. *Professional and Popular Medicine in France, 1770–1830.* Cambridge: Cambridge University Press, 1988.

Ramsey, Matthew. "Traditional Medicine and Medical Enlightenment: The Regulation of Secret Remedies in the Ancien Regime." *Historical Reflections/Réflections Historiques* 9, no. 1–2 (1982): 215–32.

Rausky, Franklin. *Mesmer ou la révolution thérapeutic.* Paris: Payot, 1977.

Reese, Mark. *Moshe Feldenkrais: A Life in Movement.* Vol. 1. San Rafael, CA: Reesekress Somatics, 2015.

Renberg, Gil H. *Where Dreams May Come: Incubation Sanctuaries in the Greco-Roman World.* Cambridge, MA: Harvard University Press, 2017.

Riffe, Jon. "Deleuze's Concept of Quasi-cause." In *Deleuze Studies* 11, no. 2 (2017): 278–94.

Risse, Guenter B. "Asclepius at Epidaurus: The Divine Power of Healing Dreams." Lecture, May 13, 2008. https://www.academia.edu/11379393/Asclepius_at_Epidaurus _The_Divine_Power_of_Healing.

Roosth, Sophia. *Synthetic: How Life Got Made.* Chicago: University of Chicago Press, 2017.

Root-Bernstein, Robert. "Antigenic Complementarity in the Induction of Autoimmunity: A General Theory and Review." *Autoimmunity Reviews* 76 no. 5 (2007): 272–77.

Rošker, Jana S. "The Concept of *Qi* in Chinese Philosophy: A Vital Force of Cosmic and Human Breath." In *Atmospheres of Breathing,* edited by Lenart Škof and Petri Berndtson, 127–40. Albany: State University of New York Press, 2018.

Roussillon, René. *Du baquet de Mesmer au "baquet" de Freud: Une archéologie du cadre et de les pratique psychoanaltiques.* Paris: Presses Universitaires de France, 1992.

Savitt, Todd. *Race and Medicine in Nineteenth- and Twentieth-Century America.* Kent, OH: Kent State University Press, 2007.

Schrödinger, Erwin. *What Is Life? The Physical Aspect of the Living Cell.* Cambridge: Cambridge University Press, 1944.

Shapin, Steven. "Descartes the Doctor: Rationalism and Its Therapies." *British Journal for the History of Science* 33, no. 116, pt. 2 (2000): 131–54.

Shapiro, Arthur, and Elaine Shapiro. *The Powerful Placebo: From Ancient Priest to Modern Physician.* Baltimore: Johns Hopkins University Press, 1997.

Shepard, Michael, and Norman Sartorius, eds. *Non-specific Aspects of Treatment.* Toronto: Hans Huber, 1989.

Sigerest, Henry. "History of Medicine and the History of Science." *Bulletin of the Institute of the History of Medicine* 4, no. 1 (1936): 1–13.

Silverstein, Arthur. "Horror Autotoxicus versus Autoimmunity: The Struggle for Recognition." *Nature Immunology* 2, no. 4 (2001): 279–81.

Simondon, Gilbert. *L'individuation psychic et collective: À la lumière des notions de forme, information, potentiel et métastabilité.* Paris: Aubier, 1987.

Simondon, Gilbert. *L'individu et sa genèse physico-biologique.* Grenoble, France: Jérome Millon, 1995.

Škof, Lenart, and Petri Berndtson, eds. *Atmospheres of Breathing.* Albany: State University of New York Press, 2018.

Slatman, Jenny. "Transparent Bodies: Revealing the Myth of Interiority." In *The Body Within: Art, Medicine and Visualization,* edited by Renée van de Vall and Robert Zwijnenberg, 107–22. Leiden: Brill, 2009.

Sontag, Susan. *"Illness as Metaphor" and "AIDS and Its Metaphors."* New York: Picador, 2001.

Spinoza, Baruch. *Ethics.* Translated by Edwin Curley. London: Penguin, 1994 [1677].

Spiro, Howard. *Doctors, Patients, and Placebos.* New Haven, CT: Yale University Press, 1986.

Staden, Pieter van. "Jesus and Asklepios." *Ekklesiastikos Pharos* 80, no. 1 (1998): 84–111.

Starr, Paul. *The Social Transformation of American Medicine.* New York: Basic Books, 1982.

Steger, Florian, Margot M. Saar, and Franz Steiner Verlag. *Asclepius: Medicine and Cult.* Stuttgart: Franz Steiner Verlag, 2018.

Stengers, Isabelle. "The Doctor and the Charlatan." In *Doctors and Healers,* by Isabelle Stengers and Tobie Nathan, translated by Stephen Muecke, 87–132. Cambridge: Polity, 2018.

Stengers, Isabelle. *The Invention of Modern Science.* Translated by Daniel W. Smith. Minneapolis: University of Minnesota Press, 2000.

Stiegler, Bernard. *Disbelief and Discredit.* Vol. 1, *The Decadence of Industrial Democracies.* Translated by Daniel Ross and Suzanne Arnold. London: Polity, 2011.

Stiegler, Bernard. *Technics and Time.* Vol. 1, *The Fault of Epimetheus.* Translated by Richard Beardsworth and George Collins. Stanford, CA: Stanford University Press, 1998.

Stiegler, Bernard. *What Makes Life Worth Living? On Pharmacology.* Translated by Daniel Ross. London: Polity, 2013.

Suzuki, Shunryu. *Zen Mind, Beginner's Mind.* 40th anniversary ed. Boston: Shambala, 2010.

Sweet, Victoria. *God's Hotel: A Doctor, a Hospital, and a Pilgrimage to the Heart of Medicine.* New York: Riverhead, 2012.

Sweet, Victoria. "Hildegard of Bingen and the Greening of Medieval Medicine." *Bulletin of the History of Medicine* 73, no. 3 (1999): 381–403.

Sweet, Victoria. *Rooted in the Earth, Rooted in the Sky: Hildegard of Bingen and Premodern Medicine*. New York: Routledge, 2006.

Sweet, Victoria. *Slow Medicine: The Way to Healing*. New York: Riverhead, 2017.

Treichler, Paula. "AIDS, Homophobia, and Biomedical Discourse: Epidemic of Signification." *October* 43 (1987): 31–70.

Treichler, Paula. *How to Have Theory in an Epidemic: Cultural Chronicles of AIDS*. Durham, NC: Duke University Press, 1999.

Turner, Kelly A. *Radical Remission: Surviving Cancer against All Odds*. New York: HarperOne, 2014.

van der Eijk, Philip J. "Aristotle's Psycho-physiological Account of the Body-Soul Relationship." In *Psyche and Soma: Physicians and Metaphysicians on the Mind-Body Problem from Antiquity to Enlightenment*, edited by John P. Wright and Paul Potter, 57–78. Oxford: Clarendon, 2000.

van der Eijk, Philip J. *Medicine and Philosophy in Classical Antiquity: Doctors and Philosophers on Nature, Soul, Health and Disease*. Cambridge: Cambridge University Press, 2005.

van der Eijk, Philip J. "The 'Theology' of the Hippocratic Treatise *On the Sacred Disease*." In *Medicine and Philosophy in Classical Antiquity: Doctors and Philosophers on Nature, Soul, Health and Disease*, 45–73. Cambridge: Cambridge University Press, 2005.

Veaumorel, M. Caullet de. *Aphorismes de M. Mesmer*. 3rd ed. Paris: M. Quinquet, 1785.

Vengi, E., Daniela Gilardi, Stefanos Bonovas, Bianca E. Corrò, Julia Menichetti, Daniela Leone, Allocca Mariangela, Federica Furfaro, Silvio Danese, and Gionata Fiorino. "Illness Perception in Inflammatory Bowel Disease Patients Is Different between Patients with Active Disease or in Remission: A Prospective Cohort Study." *Journal of Crohn's and Colitis* 13, no. 4 (2019): 417–23.

Vernadsky, Vladimir. *The Biosphere*. Translated by David Langmuir. New York: Copernicus, 1997.

Vernant, Jean-Pierre. *Myth and Society in Ancient Greece*. Translated by Janet Lloyd. New York: Zone, 1990.

Vernant, Jean-Pierre. *Myth and Thought among the Greeks*. Translated by Janet Lloyd with Jeff Fort. New York: Zone, 2006.

Vernant, Jean-Pierre, and Pierre Vidal-Naquet. *Myth and Tragedy in Ancient Greece*. Translated by Janet Lloyd. New York: Zone, 1988.

Watney, Simon. *Policing Desire: Pornography, AIDS and the Media*. Minneapolis: University of Minnesota Press, 1996.

Watts, Geoff. *Pleasing the Patient: A New Agenda for Medicine*. London: Faber and Faber, 1992.

Whitehead, Alfred North. *The Function of Reason: Louis Clark Vanuxem Foundation Lectures*. Princeton, NJ: Princeton University Press, 1929.

Wickkiser, Bronwen L. *Asklepios, Medicine, and the Politics of Healing in Fifth-Century Greece: Between Craft and Cult*. Baltimore: Johns Hopkins University Press, 2008.

Wilcox, Bruce, and Rita Colwell. "Emerging and Reemerging Infectious Diseases: Biocomplexity as an Interdisciplinary Paradigm." *EcoHealth* 2, no. 4 (2005): 244–57.

Winnicott, Donald W. "Mind and Its Relation to the Psyche-Soma." *British Journal of Medical Psychology* 27, no. 4 (1954): 201–9.

Winnicott, Donald W. *Playing and Reality*. London: Tavistock, 1971.

Winnicott, Donald W. "Psychosomatic Illness in Its Positive and Negative Aspects." *International Journal of Psychoanalysis* 47, no. 4 (1966): 510–16.

Yoo, Brian B., and Sarkis K. Masmanian. "The Enteric Network: Interactions between the Immune and Nervous Systems of the Gut." *Immunity* 46, no. 6 (2017): 910–26.

# Index

family, 13, 49–51, 74–75, 138; Jewish, 70–71,
   97–98; of patients, 58–59; values, 20, 24,
   82, 86–87
Farman, Abou, 168n61
father, 20, 50–51, 67
Feldenkrais, Moshe, 121, 124–33, 137, 140,
   159–60, 178n65, 184nn7–9
feminism, 38, 83, 187n42
Ferrucci, Piero, 135
fevers, 19
Ficino, Marsilio, 24
flaring (acute Crohn's episode), 17–18
Flexner, Abraham, 88–90, 92–93, 95, 97, 105
Flexner Report. See Bulletin Number Four
   (Flexner; Flexner Report)
"folk medicine," 13
for-profit institutions, 87–88, 165n38
Foucault, Michel, 10, 54, 103, 167n46, 168n57,
   186n33; on governance, 57–58; on life/
   living, 190n77, 190n79, 191n83; on subju-
   gated knowledge, 16, 118–10; on thinking,
   42–43, 69, 75–76
France, 104–14. See also royal commission,
   French
Francis (Pope), 161–62
Frank, Arthur, 36, 42, 69
Franklin, Benjamin, 109, 110, 113
freedom, 43, 128
Freud, Sigmund, 97–100, 128, 145, 175n38,
   176–77nn41–44, 177nn46–47, 177n51,
   184n7, 189n70
Functional Integration (Feldenkrais
   Method), 126–27

Gabor, Zsa Zsa, 59
Galenic/Aristotelian tradition, 25, 105
Galenic/Hippocratic tradition, 22, 105, 157,
   174n25, 192nn94–95
gastroenterology/gastroenterologists, 11,
   18–19, 67, 70, 171n43; diagnostic testing by,
   51–52; relationships with, 74–77
gastrointestinal tract, 62–63, 170n27
gay men, 12, 19, 78, 122
gay-related immune deficiency. See GRID
gender, 39, 71
genetics, 29, 62, 64, 71–72, 174n32
Georgetown University, 75–76, 122
germ theory of disease, 91–95, 173n22

Ginzburg, Leon, 61
global warming, 8
God, 25, 104, 165n6
God's Hotel (Sweet), 4
going-on-living, 7–9, 14–15, 35, 38, 81, 143,
   145, 164n22
Gonzalo (friend), 2
governance/governability, 53, 57, 79; medical,
   58, 88, 164n35
graduate school, 122, 134–35
Graham, Martha, 124
gravity, 36, 106, 127
Greece, ancient, 56–57
greenness/greening. See viriditas (greenness/
   greening)
GRID (gay-related immune deficiency), 78
growth/growing, 4, 7, 9
guided imagery therapy, 99–102, 115, 118–19,
   123, 128, 185n14
Guillotin, Joseph-Ignace, 109
gut (enteric nervous system), 62–63, 77–78,
   102
gut-brain-microbiome axis, 73, 102

Halprin, Anna, 124
Haraway, Donna, 171n46
Harmonic Convergence (astrological event),
   133–34
Harper, Susan, 138–39, 146, 149, 187n41
Healer's Art (college course), 84, 176n39
healing. See specific topics
healing power of nature. See vis medicatrix
   naturae
health. See specific topics
health insurance, 21, 51, 82, 96, 128–29, 149,
   172n6
heredity, 71–72
hierarchies, 90, 111–12
higher education, 89
high school, 74–75, 183n2
Hildegard of Bingen, 4–5, 22, 160
Hippocrates, 31, 39, 55
Hippocratic/Galenic tradition. See Galenic/
   Hippocratic tradition
Hippocratic oath, 22, 155
hip replacement, 11–12, 164n34
history, 12–13, 22, 42, 117, 172n5, 192n94
HIV/AIDS. See AIDS/HIV

Holm, Hanya, 124
homeostasis, 26, 166n8
Hoover Pavilion, Stanford University Hospital, 19–21, 78
hormones, 22–23
*horror autotoxicus*, 65, 170n36
hospitals/hospitalization, 39, 44–45, 58–59, 81; ICUs in, 2, 19–29. *See also specific hospitals*
host organisms, 91–92, 174n25, 174n28, 176n43
humans, 8–9, 63, 129, 175n37; capacities of, 13, 124, 127–28, 140, 145, 151
Hume, David, 104
*humidium radicale* (radical moisture), 5
Humira (medication), 18, 60–61, 169n18
humors/humoralism, 4–5, 26
hylomorphism, 142, 188n56
hypotheses, testable, 111

ICUs, hospital, 2, 19–29
identity/identities, 70, 71–72, 86, 154, 159
ignorance, 9–11, 14, 30–31, 157
illness/illnesses, 26, 106; diseases *versus*, 35–36, 95; as experience, 34–36, 41
imagination, 73, 96, 121, 127, 178n65, 181n109; guided imagery therapy and, 99–102, 115, 118–19, 123, 128; knowledge vs., 68–69; medical, 25, 37–38, 68–69, 103; placebo effect and, 115–18; power of, 100–102, 104–5, 115–19; royal commission on, 111–14, 180n104
immaterialism, 98
immunity/immune system, 63–65, 92–93, 174n25, 174n28
immunodeficiency, 64, 65–66
immunological tolerance phenomena, 64
immunology, 27, 63–64, 97–98, 153
immunosuppression, 18, 66, 145
imperialism, 27
inanimate beings, 8–9
inborn heat. See *calor inatus* (inborn heat)
*In Cold Blood* (movie), 59
incontinence, 15; adolescent, 17–18, 49–52, 74–75
indeterminacy/indetermination, 8, 10, 29
indigenous therapies, 13

individuality/individualism, 131–32, 140, 146–47
individuation, 132, 142–44, 145, 148–49, 188n51, 189n67, 189n69
industries, 117; pharmaceutical, 27–28, 32, 169–70nn18–19
inexplicable healing/recovery, 4, 5
infants, 15, 40, 127, 129, 137, 145, 184n13
infections, 6, 19–20, 91
infectious diseases, 27, 91, 94–95, 175n37
inflammation, Crohn's disease causing, 17–18, 53, 61–62, 66–70
inflammatory bowel diseases, 41 , 59, 70, 102–3, 177n59; open-label placebos for, 118, 182n121
injuries, 7–8
innate vigor. See *phusis* (innate vigor)
inoculation, 91, 173n22
intelligence, 30, 38, 47
interior world (*milieu intérieur*), 26
interleukin-17A, 60–61, 66
internal resonance, 141, 144, 146, 148–50, 188n51, 191n86
internists, 51
interpretation, medical, 53–54, 73
*Interpretation of Dreams, The* (Freud), 97
intestinal obstruction, 18
*Introduction à l'étude de médecine expérimentale* (Bernard), 26
intuition, 28–29
investments in knowledge, 30–31
isolation, 81

James, William, 87, 98
Janowitz, Henry (Dr. J.), 61–62, 68
Jenner, Edward, 173n22
Jerne, Niels, 174n28
Jewish people/ancestry, 20, 70–71, 82, 97–98, 132; Crohn's prevalent in, 52, 71–72
Joann (therapist), 83
Joliot-Curie, Frédéric, 125, 133
Joliot-Curie, Irène, 125, 133
Jones, Bill T., 164n33
*Journal of the American Medical Association*, 61, 117
judgment, 35, 55
Jullien, François, 190n80

Jung, Carl, 98, 100, 176nn41–42
Jussieu, Antoine-Laurent de, 109–10

Kano, Jigoro, 125
Kant, Immanuel, 104
Kerényi, Carl, 157–58
Kesey, Ken, 2, 124
Kitchen Table Wisdom (Remen), 84
knowledge, 9–10, 39, 55, 68, 103, 141, 178n64;
   biomedical, 100; bioscientific, 11, 28–30,
   93; as distinct from learning, 14–15; of
   doctors, 30–31, 55–57; scientific, 11–12, 47,
   86, 90; subjugated, 16, 118–19, 153; thera-
   peutic power of, 33, 39, 55, 69–70, 157.
   See also limitations; medical knowledge
Koch, Robert, 90–91, 94, 175nn33–34
Kronos (Greek Titan), 49, 168n1

laboratory-based practices, 90–94
Lacan, Jacques, 30
Laguna Honda Hospital, 6
Lamarck, Jean-Baptiste, 72
language, 53–54, 151–53, 182n111; war-
   centered, 27, 37, 92. See also etymology;
   names/naming
Lavoisier, Antoine, 107–8, 109, 112, 114
law of noncontradiction, 39, 65, 148
laws/legality, 11, 72, 88, 186n37
learning to heal, 1–3, 9, 14–15, 38, 121, 130–32,
   159–60; Continuum approach to, 138–39;
   Feldenkrais Method and, 123–28, 185n19;
   modern medicine impacting, 12–13; neuromuscular, 124, 127–28, 136–37, 145
lesbians, 83
leukemia, 58
Leyden jar, 106
licensure, medical, 54, 88
life/living, 4–5, 7, 9, 10, 79, 132, 140, 144,
   164n18; Bergson on, 8, 34, 36; bodies,
   24–25; death and, 37–38; Foucault on,
   190n77, 190n79, 191n83
life sciences, 10, 164n22
life support, 69, 81
limitations, 12, 28, 48, 65–66, 157, 162; of
   bioscientific knowledge, 29–30, 93; of
   medical knowledge, 23–24, 67–68, 76–77;
   of medical thinking, 41–42; of scientific
   medicine, 99

lived spirituality, 146–47
liver, 19
Los Angeles, California, 135–36, 138
Louis XVI (monarch), 104, 106, 109–10,
   181n109

magicians/magic, 57, 97
management, medicine as, 20, 22, 53
Marcuse, Herbert, 139
marijuana, 77–78, 171n50
marketing, medical, 56, 60–61
Marxism, 20, 121, 185n14
Maryland, 2, 71, 74–75
materialism, 20, 24, 85
mathematics, 108–8
measurability, 32–33, 115–18
mechanical reductionism, 23–28
medical: education, 4, 87–90, 92–93, 95–96,
   105, 173n16, 176n40; governance, 58, 88,
   164n35; imagination, 25. See also testing,
   medical
medical-industrial complex, 45
medical knowledge, 12–15, 90, 102, 158–59;
   authority of, 78–79; of doctors, 7, 30–31;
   healing curtailed by, 67–68; limits of,
   23–24, 67–68, 76–77; medical education
   and, 87–88
medications, 11, 53; profitability of, 54–55,
   60–61; toxicity of, 14, 20, 66–68; withdrawal from, 20, 67–68, 83–86. See also
   specific medications
medicine. See specific topics
medieval medicine, 5
Meditations on First Philosophy (Descartes),
   25
Medline (database), 21–22
Mendocino, California, 133–34
mental illnesses, 35–36, 73–74
Merleau-Ponty, Maurice, 141
Mesmer, Franz Anton, 104–10, 179n73,
   179n86, 183n123
mesmerism, 104–13, 179n73, 179n87
Mesmer ou la révolution thérapeutic (Rausky),
   180n104
metaphors, 25, 54, 72, 92, 98–99, 133, 161,
   169n5, 169n7; allergies as, 60, 65, 70
metaphysics, 24, 29, 141, 148, 188n53
metastability, 142–43

Metchnikoff, Élie, 65, 92–93, 174nn24–25, 174nn28–29, 176n43

microbes, 62–64, 90–94. *See also* bacteria

micromovements, 136–37

middle-class, 82, 149

*milieu extérieur* (exterior world), 26

*milieu intérieur* (interior world), 26

mind, 40–41, 130

"Mind and Its Relation to the Psyche-Soma" (Winnicott), 40

mind/body dualism, 123, 130, 137, 181n104, 187n44

modern dance, 124–25

modern medicine, 7, 12–13, 44, 87, 118–19, 153–58, 162; in medical education, 88–90, 92–93

modern science, 68, 103

Moerman, Daniel, 182n115

monoclonal antibodies, 60–61, 66

morality, 58–59

mother, 67, 75, 76

movement/motion, 34, 187n43; ATM as, 124–28, 159; Continuum approach to, 135–41, 143, 145–46, 149–50, 152, 155; tai chi as, 132–34

music, 20–21

*My Grandfather's Blessings* (Remen), 84

mysteries, 4, 5, 32–33, 86

Nagel, Thomas, 34

names/naming, 55, 159, 170n21; in diagnoses, 51–53; of experiences, 34, 83

Naomi. *See* Remen, Rachel (Naomi)

narrative medicine, 96, 176n39

National Center for Complementary and Integrative Health, 165n41, 183n122

Native Americans, 4, 5–7

nature, 5, 9, 30, 32, 92, 108, 111, 163n14

near-death experiences, 1, 21, 45, 73, 86, 147

neuromuscular learning/capacities, 124, 127–28, 136–37, 145

neuroreceptors, 62, 77–78

neurotransmitters, 62

New Age, 147, 152

"New Method of Healing, A" (Assagioli lecture), 99

Newton, Isaac, 106, 172n5

New York City, 71

*New York Times, The,* 161

Nietzsche, Friedrich, 7, 49, 166n15

Nikolais, Alwin, 124

Nobel Prize, 65

"nocebo," 182n120

noncontradiction, law of, 39, 65, 148

nonmedical staff, hospital, 39

nonrepeatable experiences, 32–33

non-Western practices, 98, 133, 166n12

*Normal and the Pathological, The* (Canguilhem), 35

North America, 12, 87–89

not-knowing, 14, 31, 49, 86–87, 157–58

not-self/self paradigm, 63–65

novels, death in, 59

nurses, 19, 39, 58, 74, 81, 86, 162

objectivity, 34, 114–17

O'Hair, Madalyn Murray, 20

*Omphale* (houseboat), 84–85

oncology/oncologists, 13–14, 33

*One Flew over the Cuckoo's Nest* (Kesey), 2

*On Kissing, Tickling and Being Bored* (Phillips), 172n4

*On the Origin of Species* (Darwin), 72

ontological theory of diseases, 46–47

open-label placebos, 118, 182n121

Oppenheimer, Gordon, 61

*Oprah* (television show), 83

organisms, 7, 24, 91–92, 174n25, 185n28; Bernard on, 25–26; Descartes on, 25, 184n4

organ systems, 63

outcomes, therapeutic, 32, 118

out-of-body experiences, 19, 21, 146

painkillers, 18, 19

pain management, 20

palliative care, 13

Palo Alto, California, 1, 81

pandemics, 12, 161–62

Paracelsus, 24

paradigms, 94–95, 131, 140–41; self/not-self, 63–65; *vis medicatrix naturae* as, 26–27

paradoxes, 41, 68–69; of autoimmune etiologies, 71

paralysis, 137

parasites, 91–92

parents, 49–51, 67–68, 70 , 82

Pasteur, Louis, 90–92, 173n22, 174n29
Pasteur Institute, 27
pathogen-disease correlations, 94–95
pathogens. *See* bacteria
pathological anatomy, 37, 46, 88
pathology, 11, 35, 47, 61, 90–94; disease as, 44–45
patients, 44–46, 81–82, 86, 95, 164n35, 176n39; animal magnetism treatment for, 105–14, 180n93; doctor relationships with, 53, 96
pedagogies, 130, 132, 168n57, 173n16
pediatricians, 51, 75
performance principle, 139, 187n47
Pert, Candace, 187n44
pharmaceutical industry, 27–28, 32, 169–70nn18–19
pharmacopoeia, 5, 26, 57
PhD studies, 18, 76–77
phenomena, 10, 46, 54, 64, 87, 103, 150, 170n37; gastrointestinal, 62
philanthropy, 173n15
Phillips, Adam, 172n4
*phusis* (innate vigor), 5, 188n53, 193n100
*Physica and Causae et Curae* (Hildegard), 4
physicians. *See* doctors
physics, 90, 113, 142, 181n107
*Picture Mommy Dead* (movie), 59
Pindar, 193n106
placebos/placebo effect, 115–18, 158, 180n102, 182n113, 182n115, 182n120; open-label, 118, 182n121
Planet Art Network, 133
plants. *See* nature
Plato, 103, 146
play, 150–51, 169n7, 190n82, 191n84
pleasure, 115–16, 137–38
poison. *See* toxicity of medications
political values, 7, 12, 135
population model of disease, 167n35
possibility/possibilities, 7, 10, 33, 41, 136, 149
post-truth, 32
potential/potentialities, 9, 99, 142–43; healing, 102, 119, 141, 158; imagination and, 118–19; profitability, 32
*Potent Self, The* (Feldenkrais), 184n8
power, 8–9, 96, 100, 138, 172n8; of imagination, 100–102, 104–5, 115–19; of medical

knowledge, 68; of medicine, 57, 69, 78. *See also* therapeutic power of knowledge; *vis medicatrix naturae* (healing power of nature)
"Powerful Placebo, The" (Beecher), 117
predictability, 33, 46
prednisone, 18–19, 70, 78, 171n40; during adolescence, 22–23, 66–68, 73–76; withdrawal from, 67–68, 83
preindividual, 142–44, 148, 150, 189n67, 191n82
premodern medicine, 4–5
prescriptions, 39, 53, 59, 75, 162, 164n32; for prednisone, 18–19, 66
Pritchett, Henry, 89–90, 96–97
probability, 33, 167n27
professional authority, 87–88
profitability, 32, 136, 139; of medical educations, 87; of medications, 54–55, 60–61; of vaccines, 27, 91
prognosis/prognoses, 33, 56, 78–79
*Prognostic* (Hippocrates), 56
protocols, 44, 87, 94, 107–13, 116–17, 158, 175n34
proto-queerness, 68, 75, 145
psyche, 40–41, 98, 189n69
psychiatry, 13
psychoanalysis, 96–98, 145, 172n4, 176n41
psychology/psychological, 67, 83–86, 96
psychoneuroimmunology, 171n43, 178n60, 182n116
psychosocial dimension, 128–30, 146, 171n42, 184n13
psychosomatic illnesses, 41
psychosynthesis, 96–100, 176n41
psychotherapy, 67–68, 82, 98, 135
public health, 13, 27, 94, 106–10, 175n34
public school, 74

quarantines, 27, 175n34
questions, 13–14, 23, 103–4

race, 39, 171n52
radical healing experiences, 17, 24, 33, 45–46, 131, 149
radical moisture (*humidium radicale*), 5
rationality/rationalism, 65, 105, 113, 118–19, 158–59, 181n107, 183n123, 192n99

steroids, 18–20, 66; during adolescence,
22–23, 73–75
Stiegler, Bernard, 189n68
stigmas, social, 1, 74
striving (*conatus*), 7, 163n12
subjectivity, 34, 129, 191n82
subject/object dichotomy, 139–40
subjects, 30–31, 40, 110, 123, 166n15, 186n30;
experimental, 111–13; patients as, 44–46
subjugated knowledge, 16, 118–19, 153
suffering, 40, 44–46, 55–56, 70
Supreme Court, US, 172n8
surgery, 19–21, 26, 57, 61, 82, 170n23
survival, 6, 33
Sweet, Victoria, 4–7, 168n49
symptoms, 11, 41, 44; cholera, 94; Crohn's
disease, 1, 61, 70–71; interpretation of,
53–54; pathological anatomy and, 37, 46;
suppression of, 66; testing correlating, 53.
*See also specific symptoms*
syphilis, 171n52

tai chi, 132–34, 149, 159
Tarde, Gabriel, 98
teaching, 43, 84, 89
teaching hospitals, 52
technologies, 90–91, 106; biotechnologies,
62–63; public health, 10, 27; vaccines as,
91–92, 173nn22–23
tendencies, 36, 79, 147, 149; toward anxiety,
49–50; toward death, 47; healing, 20–21,
37–39, 47; hereditary, 71–72; individualizing, 131–32
Terry (patient), 4, 5–7
testicular cancer, 36
testing, medical, 19, 53, 59–60, 77–78; blind-
testing for, 112–15, 183n123; blood work as,
51–52, 77; double-blind testing as, 116–17,
180n102, 183n123. *See also* placebos/pla-
cebo effect
Theosophy, 98, 177n49
therapeutic power of knowledge, 33, 39, 55,
69–70, 157
therapeutics, 13, 54–55, 57, 61–62, 158–59,
183n122; biomedicine and, 167n35; humoralist, 26–27; limits of, 65–66; reductionism curtailing, 24; scientific assessment of,
107–17. *See also specific therapies*

thermodynamics, 36–37
thinking/thought, 54; Foucault on, 42–43,
69, 75–76; medical, 41–42, 45
*Three Essays on the Theory of Sexuality*
(Freud), 97
time/temporality, 6, 55–56, 85, 151–52, 191n85
toilet training, 15, 50, 165n36, 184n13
toxicity of medications, 14, 20, 66–68
training, medical, 12, 87–89, 95, 97–99,
173n16
trances (state), 20–21, 42, 86, 146–47
transformations/transformative, 4, 42,
87–88, 128–29
transindividuation, 132, 144, 146–52, 190n82,
191n86
transpersonal psychology, 96
traumas, 123, 145
treatments, medical, 11, 12, 52, 61–62
trees, 3, 146
Treichler, Paula, 161
trials, clinical, 32
*Tron* (movie), 18
true/false dichotomy, 103, 141
trust, 30, 32
truth, 23, 43, 103, 119, 141, 178n64; disqualification and, 15–16, 158; medicine and, 73,
113–14; scientific, 32, 107–8
tumor necrosis factor inhibitors, 60–61, 66
Tuskegee Institute, 171n52
Typhoid Mary, 175n34

ulcerative colitis, 59
uncertainty, 33, 65–66
unconscious, 99, 130
unhappiness, 145, 177n44
unintended consequences, 29
United States (US), 13, 23, 82, 87, 136, 161,
171n52; medical education in, 88–89
Université de Paris, 105
University of Maryland hospital, 51, 58, 75

vaccines, 27, 91, 166n13, 173nn22–23
validity, scientific, 107–10
values, 7–9, 43, 129, 136–37, 145, 149, 169n4,
187n42; familial, 20, 24, 82, 86–87;
judgment, 35; medical education instilled,
88–89; political, 7, 12, 135
Vernadsky, Vladimir, 8

Vienna, Austria, 97
*viriditas* (greenness/greening), 5–7, 77–78, 134, 151
viruses, 175n34
*vis medicatrix naturae* (healing power of nature), 5, 7, 22; Bernard displacing, 26–27; modern medicine replacing, 92
vital force (*élan vital*), 29, 36
vital function, 22–23, 128–29
vitalism/vitalists, 24, 27, 29, 157, 166n21
vital values, 7–9, 169n4
vivisection, 90
vulnerability, 6, 70, 171n46

walks/walking, 127, 137, 184n11
warfare, language of, 27, 37, 92
water, 94, 175n37
Wavy Gravy (poet), 134, 186n36
weight gain, 66–67, 74
weight loss, 70–71

Western ontotheology, 141–42, 188n55
Western thinking/thought, 12–13, 24, 103, 133, 141–42, 190n80
Whitehead, Alfred North, 9, 75–76
wind-person (imaginary figure), 100–101, 145
Winnicott, Donald, 40–41, 150, 190n82
withdrawal from medications, 20, 67–68, 83–86
Wolfe, Tom, 2
women's medicine, 13
working class, 111–12
workshops, 128, 135, 139; Continuum, 141, 149–50, 152
World Health Organization, 94

X-rays, 51

Zen Buddhism, 31
Zeus (Greek god), 168n1, 193n106
Zürich, Switzerland, 97